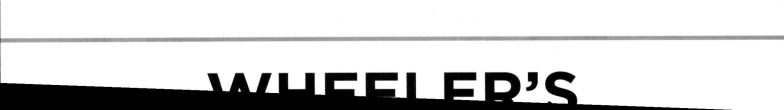

WHEELER'S

ELEVENTH EDITION

WHEELER'S

DENTAL ANATOMY, PHYSIOLOGY, AND OCCLUSION

STANLEY J. NELSON, DDS, MS

Professor
School of Dental Medicine
University of Nevada
Las Vegas, Nevada

ELSEVIER

Elsevier
3251 Riverport Lane
St. Louis, Missouri 63043

WHEELER'S DENTAL ANATOMY, PHYSIOLOGY, AND OCCLUSION,
ELEVENTH EDITION

ISBN: 978-0-323-63878-4

Notice

Previous editions copyrighted 2015, 2010, 2003, 1993, 1984, 1974, 1965, 1958, 1950, and 1940.

International Standard Book Number: 978-0-323-63878-4

Content Strategist: Alexandra Mortimer
Senior Content Development Manager: Luke Held
Senior Content Development Specialist: Jennifer Wade
Publishing Services Manager: Julie Eddy
Book Production Specialist: Clay S. Broeker
Design Direction: Patrick Ferguson

Printed in Canada

Last digit is the print number: 9 8 7 6 5 4 3 2 1

Working together
to grow libraries in
developing countries

www.elsevier.com • www.bookaid.org

This edition is dedicated to my father,
Charles S. Nelson, DDS

Preface

It is hard for me to realize that this eleventh edition of *Wheeler's Dental Anatomy, Physiology, and Occlusion* marks my career of over 40 years in dental education and practice. It is overwhelming how quickly the time has passed. While the practice of dentistry has changed greatly over this time, my experience and passion for teaching have not so much. I consider myself to have been blessed with the chance to work so long with eager, bright, highly motivated, and dedicated students of dentistry. Previous editions of this book have been translated in seven languages that I know of, and it doesn't seem to matter which country these students live in or what stage of their career they are in; learning is the driving goal for them, and watching them reach understanding in what I was trying to teach energizes me to this day. The passion for learning is the reason for the eleventh edition, and I hope this book helps students of dentistry achieve the knowledge they work so hard for.

Many have contributed to this eleventh edition of *Wheeler's Dental Anatomy, Physiology, and Occlusion*. I thank my colleague Dr. Eve Chung for her help in updating many of the illustrations to color photographs. I also need to recognize the previous contributions from my colleagues: Dr. Edward Herschaft in forensic odontology (Chapter 4), Dr. Wendy Woodall in restorative dentistry (Chapter 17), Dr. Larry Zoller and Dr. Josh Polanski in head and neck anatomy and neurology (Chapters 14 and 15), Dr. Owen Sanders and Dr. Cody Hughes in pediatric dentistry (Chapter 3), and Dr. Neamat Hassan in dental materials science and pulpal anatomy (Chapter 13). A sincere thank you to the students of the University of Nevada School of Dental Medicine for their suggestions and feedback. Special thanks to Anna Miller, Alexandra Mortimer, Luke Held, Kathleen Nahm, Jennifer Wade, Clay Broeker, and the staff of Elsevier. Lastly, of course, thank you to my wife Mary Sarah Brady for all your help and support.

To quote Dr. Wheeler from the first edition's preface: "No successful practitioner fails to recognize the importance of the fundamental form of the teeth, their alignment and their occlusion, as a basic subject serving as a background for all phases of dental practice." Thanks to all who contributed to this textbook. Thanks to all for helping improve dentistry.

SJN

Contents

1

Introduction to Dental Anatomy

LEARNING OBJECTIVES

1. Correctly define and pronounce the nomenclature (terms) as emphasized in the bold type in this and each following chapter.
2. Be able to identify each tooth of the primary and permanent dentitions using the Universal, Palmer, and Fédération Dentaire Internationale (FDI) systems.
3. Correctly name and identify the surfaces, ridges, and anatomic landmarks of each tooth.
4. Understand and describe the methods used to measure anterior and posterior teeth.
5. Learn the tables of measurements and be able to discuss size comparisons between the teeth from any viewing angle. A useful skill at this point is to start illustrating the individual teeth with line drawings.

Pretest Questions

1. The dental formula for the permanent human dentition is which of the following?
   A. I 2/2 C 1/1 M 2/2 = 10
   B. I 2/2 C 1/1 P 1/1 M 2/2 = 12
   C. I 2/2 C 1/1 P 2/2 M 2/2 = 14
   D. I 2/2 C 1/1 P 2/2 M 3/3 = 16
2. The notation for the primary mandibular left canine is which of the following according to the FDI system?
   A. 53
   B. 63
   C. 73
   D. 83
3. The notation for the primary maxillary left lateral incisor is which of the following according to the Universal system?
   A. D
   B. G
   C. E
   D. F
4. Which of the following represents the name of the bone of the tooth socket that firmly fixes each tooth root?
   A. Alveolar process
   B. Alveolus
   C. Cementoenamel junction
   D. Dentinoenamel junction

5. Which of the following terms represents the surface of a tooth that is facing toward an adjoining tooth in the same dental arch?
   A. Occlusal
   B. Incisal
   C. Facial
   D. Proximal

For additional study resources, please visit Expert Consult.

Dental anatomy is defined here as, but is not limited to, the study of the development, morphology, function, and identity of each of the teeth in the human dentitions, as well as the way in which the teeth relate in shape, form, structure, color, and function to the other teeth in the same dental arch and to the teeth in the opposing arch. Thus the study of dental anatomy, physiology, and occlusion provides one of the basic components of the skills needed to practice all phases of dentistry.

The application of dental anatomy to clinical practice can be envisioned in Fig. 1.1A, where a faulty crown form has resulted in esthetic and periodontal problems that may be corrected by an appropriate restorative dental treatment, such as that illustrated in Fig. 1.1B. The practitioner must have knowledge of the morphology, occlusion, esthetics, phonetics, and functions of these teeth to undertake such treatment.

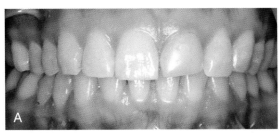
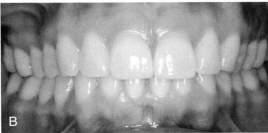

• **Fig. 1.1** Restoration of maxillary central incisors with porcelain veneers taking into account esthetics, occlusion, and periodontal health. (Case and photographs courtesy of Michael P. Webberson, DDS, Las Vegas, NV.)

Formation of the Dentitions (Overview)

Humans have two sets of teeth in their lifetime. The first set of teeth to be seen in the mouth is the **primary** or **deciduous** dentition, which begins to form prenatally at approximately 14 weeks in utero and is completed postnatally at approximately 3 years of age. In the absence of congenital disorders, dental disease, or trauma, the first teeth in this dentition begin to appear in the oral cavity at the mean age of 6 months, and the last emerge at a mean age of 28 ± 4 months. The deciduous dentition remains intact (barring loss from dental caries or trauma) until the child is approximately 6 years of age. At approximately that time, the first **succedaneous** or **permanent** teeth begin to emerge into the mouth. The emergence of these teeth begins the **transition** or **mixed dentition period,** in which there is a mixture of deciduous and succedaneous teeth present. The transition period lasts from approximately 6 to 12 years of age and ends when all the deciduous teeth have been shed. At that time, the permanent dentition period begins. Thus the transition from the primary dentition to the permanent dentition begins with the emergence of the first permanent molars, shedding of the deciduous incisors, and emergence of the permanent incisors. The mixed dentition period is often a difficult time for the young child because of habits, missing teeth, teeth of different colors and hues, crowding of the teeth, and malposed teeth.

The permanent, or succedaneous, teeth replace the exfoliated deciduous teeth in a sequence of eruption that exhibits some variance, an important topic considered in Chapter 16.

After the shedding of the deciduous canines and molars, emergence of the permanent canines and premolars, and emergence of the second permanent molars, the permanent dentition is completed (including the roots) at approximately 14 to 15 years of age, except for the third molars, which are completed at 18 to 25 years of age. In effect, the duration of the permanent dentition period is 12 or more years. The completed permanent dentition consists of 32 teeth if none is congenitally missing, which may be the case. The development of the teeth, dentitions, and the craniofacial complex is considered in Chapter 2. The development of occlusion for both dentitions is discussed in Chapter 16.

Nomenclature

The first step in understanding dental anatomy is to learn the nomenclature, or the system of names, used to describe or classify the material included in the subject. When a significant term is used for the first time here, it is emphasized in bold. Additional terms are discussed as needed in subsequent chapters.

The term **mandibular** refers to the lower jaw, or mandible. The term **maxillary** refers to the upper jaw, or maxilla. When more than one name is used in the literature to describe something, the two most commonly used names will be used initially. After that, they may be combined or used separately, as consistent with the literature of a particular specialty of dentistry, for example, **primary** or **deciduous dentition, permanent** or **succedaneous dentition.** A good case may be made for the use of both terms. By dictionary definition,[1] the term *primary* can mean "constituting or belonging to the first stage in any process." The term *deciduous* can mean "not permanent, transitory." The same unabridged dictionary refers the reader from the definition of *deciduous tooth* to *milk tooth,* which is defined as "one of the temporary teeth of a mammal that are replaced by permanent teeth; also called *baby tooth, deciduous tooth.*" The term *primary* can indicate a first dentition, and the term *deciduous* can indicate that the first dentition is

not permanent but not unimportant. The term *succedaneous* can be used to describe a successor dentition and does not suggest permanence, whereas the term *permanent* suggests a permanent dentition, which may not be the case because of dental caries, periodontal diseases, and trauma. All four of these descriptive terms appear in the professional literature.

Formulae for Mammalian Teeth

The denomination and number of all mammalian teeth are expressed by formulae that are used to differentiate the human dentitions from those of other species. The denomination of each tooth is often represented by the initial letter in its name (e.g., I for incisor, C for canine, P for premolar, M for molar). Each letter is followed by a horizontal line and the number of each type of tooth is placed above the line for the maxilla (upper jaw) and below the line for the mandible (lower jaw). The formulae include one side only, with the number of teeth in each jaw being the same for humans.

The dental formula for the primary/deciduous teeth in humans is as follows:

$$I\frac{2}{2}C\frac{1}{1}M\frac{2}{2} = 10$$

This formula should be read as: incisors, two maxillary and two mandibular; canines, one maxillary and one mandibular; molars, two maxillary and two mandibular—or 10 altogether on one side, right or left (Fig. 1.2A).

A dental formula for the permanent human dentition is as follows:

$$I\frac{2}{2}C\frac{1}{1}P\frac{2}{2}M\frac{3}{3} = 16$$

Premolars have now been added to the formula, two maxillary and two mandibular, and a third molar has been added, one maxillary and one mandibular (see Fig. 1.2B).

Systems for scoring key morphologic traits of the permanent dentition that are used for anthropologic studies are not described here. However, a few of the morphologic traits that are used in anthropologic studies[2] are considered in later chapters (e.g., shoveling, Carabelli trait, enamel extensions, peg-shaped incisors). Some anthropologists use di_1, di_2, dc, dm_1, and dm_2 notations for the deciduous dentition and I_1, I_2, C, P_1, P_2, M_1, M_2, and M_3 for the permanent teeth. These notations are generally limited to anthropologic tables because of keyboard incompatibility.

Tooth Numbering Systems

In clinical practice, some "shorthand" system of tooth notation is necessary for recording data. Several systems are in use around the world, but only a few are considered here. In 1947 a committee of the American Dental Association (ADA) recommended the symbolic system (Zsigmondy/Palmer) as the numbering method of choice.[3] However, because of difficulties with keyboard notation of the symbolic notation system, the ADA in 1968 officially recommended the "universal" numbering system. Because of some limitations and lack of widespread use internationally, recommendations for a change sometimes are made.[4]

The **Universal** system of notation for the primary dentition uses uppercase letters for each of the primary teeth: For the maxillary teeth, beginning with the right second molar, letters A through J, and for the mandibular teeth, letters K through T, beginning with

• BOX 1.2   Method of Measuring a Posterior Tooth

(Keep the long axis of the tooth vertical.)

1. Length of Crown (Buccal)

    Measurement   { Crest of buccal cusp or cusps
                    Crest of curvature at
                    cementoenamel junction

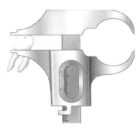

• **Fig. 1.28** Length of crown.

2. Length of Root

    Measurement   { Crest of curvature at crown cervix
                    Apex of root

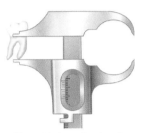

• **Fig. 1.29** Length of root.

3. Mesiodistal Diameter of Crown

    Measurement   { Crest of curvature on mesial surface
                    (mesial contact area)
                    Crest of curvature on distal surface
                    (distal contact area)

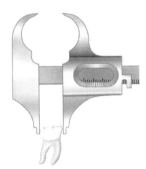

• **Fig. 1.30** Mesiodistal diameter of crown.

4. Mesiodistal Diameter of Crown at the Cervix

    Measurement   { Junction of crown and root on mesial
                    surface
                    Junction of crown and root on distal
                    surface (use caliper jaws of Boley gauge
                    instead of parallel beaks)

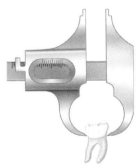

• **Fig. 1.31** Mesiodistal diameter of crown at cervix.

(Continued)

• BOX 1.2   Method of Measuring a Posterior Tooth—cont'd

5. Buccolingual Diameter of Crown

Measurement { Crest of curvature on buccal surface
Crest of curvature on lingual surface

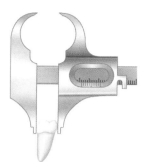

• **Fig. 1.32** Buccolingual diameter of crown.

6. Buccolingual Diameter of Crown at the Cervix

Measurement { Junction of crown and root on buccal surface
Junction of crown and root on lingual surface (use caliper jaws)

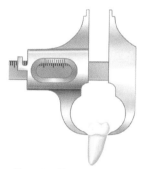

• **Fig. 1.33** Buccolingual diameter of crown at cervix.

7. Curvature of Cementoenamel Junction on Mesial

Measurement { Crest of curvature of cementoenamel junction on mesial surface
Crest of curvature of cementoenamel junction on buccal and lingual surfaces

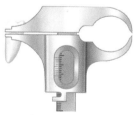

• **Fig. 1.34** Curvature of cementoenamel junction on mesial.

8. Curvature of Cementoenamel Junction on Distal
(Turn tooth around and measure as in Fig. 1.34)

Measurement { Crest of curvature of cementoenamel junction on distal surface
Crest of curvature of cementoenamel junction on buccal and lingual surfaces

Pretest Answers

1. D
2. B
3. B
4. A
5. D

References

1. *Webster's new universal unabridged dictionary.* New York, 1996, Barnes & Noble Books.
2. Turner II CG, Nichol CR, Scott GR: Scoring procedures for key morphological traits of the permanent dentition: the Arizona State University Dental Anthropology System. In Kelley MA, Larsen CS, editors: *Advances in dental anthropology*, New York, 1991, Wiley-Liss.
3. Lyons H: Committee adopts official method for the symbolic designation of teeth, *J Am Dent Assoc* 34:647, 1947.
4. Peck S, Peck L: A time for change of tooth numbering systems, *J Dent Educ* 57:643, 1993.
5. Carlsen O: *Dental morphology*, Copenhagen, 1987, Munksgaard.
6. Szentpetery J, Kormendi M: Deciduous incisors with a serrated edge, *Fogorvosi Szemle* 82(2), 1989. [Budapest].
7. Black GV: *Descriptive anatomy of the human teeth*, ed 4, Philadelphia, 1897, S.S. White Dental Manufacturing.

Bibliography

American Dental Association, Committee on Nomenclature: Committee adopts official method for the symbolic designation of teeth, *J Am Dent Assoc* 34:647, 1947.
American Dental Association, Committee on Dental Education and Hospitals: Tooth numbering and radiographic mounting, *J Am Dent Assoc Trans* 109:25–247, 1968.
Fédération Dentaire Internationale: Two-digit system of designating teeth, *Int Dent J* 21:104, 1971.
Goodman P: A universal system for identifying permanent and primary teeth, *J Dent Child* 34:312, 1987.
Haderup V: Dental nomenklatur og stenograft, *Dansk Tandl Tidskr* 3:3, 1891.
Palmer C: Palmer's dental notation, *Dental Cosmos* 33:194, 1981.
World Health Organization: *Oral health surveys: basic methods*, ed 3, Geneva, 1987, World Health Organization.
Zsigmondy A: Grundzüge einer praktischen Methode zur raschen und genauen Vonnerkung der zahnärztlichen Beobachtungen und Operationen, *Dtsch Vjschr Zahnhk* 1:209, 1861.
Zsigmondy A: A practical method for rapidly noting dental observations and operations, *Br Dent J* 17:580, 1874.

2

Development and Eruption of the Teeth

LEARNING OBJECTIVES

1. Correctly define and pronounce the new terms as emphasized in the bold type.
2. Understand prenatal, perinatal, and postnatal tooth human tooth development.
3. List and discuss average ages of initial calcification, crown completed, emergence, and root completed for the primary and permanent dentitions.

Pretest Questions

1. Which of the following teeth is not considered a succedaneous tooth (Universal system)?
   A. 24
   B. 19
   C. 28
   D. 11
2. Which of the following best represents the order of emergence of permanent teeth from earliest to latest eruption (Universal system of numbering)?
   A. 19, 8, 5, 11
   B. 8, 19, 5, 11
   C. 8, 5, 19, 11
   D. 19, 5, 11, 8
3. The dental pulp's primary function is the formation of which of the following?
   A. Enamel
   B. Dentin
   C. Cementum
   D. Periodontal ligament
4. Passage of a primary tooth crown through the alveolar gingiva occurs when approximately what fraction of the tooth root is developed?
   A. 3/4
   B. 2/3
   C. 1/2
   D. 1/4
5. Which of the following permanent teeth tend to show evidence of calcification at birth?
   A. Central incisors
   B. Canines
   C. First molar
   D. Second molar

For additional study resources, please visit Expert Consult.

Knowledge of the development of the teeth and their emergence into the oral cavity is applicable to clinical practice, anthropology, demography, forensics, and paleontology. However, dental applications are considered primarily. This chapter considers the development and eruption of the teeth, specific chronologies of both the primary and permanent human dentitions, dental age, tooth formation standards, and applications to dental practice (e.g., an understanding of both the chronology of dental development so that surgical intervention does not harm normal growth and the relationship between dental age and the effects of disease and environmental risks). The use of the terms **primary** and **deciduous**, or often, **primary/deciduous**, reflects the difference of opinion about the most appropriate term to describe the first dentition in humans. Readers of the literature are able to deal objectively with both terms.

Clinical Considerations

It must be kept in mind that the dental practitioner sees in a "normal" healthy mouth not only the **clinical crowns** of the teeth surrounded by the gingival tissues but also the number, shape, size, position, coloration, and angulations of the teeth; the outlines of the roots of the teeth; occlusal contacts; evidence of function and parafunction; and phonetics and esthetics. Most of the parts of the teeth that are hidden by the gingiva can be visualized radiographically. This can also be done by using a periodontal probe to locate the depth of normal or pathologically deepened gingival crevices or a dental explorer to sense the surfaces of the teeth within the gingival crevice apical to the free gingival margin as far as the epithelial attachment of the gingiva to the enamel. In addition, in pathologically deepened crevices, tooth surfaces can be sensed as far as the attachment of the periodontal ligament to the cementum. Perhaps the simplest example of clinical observation is the assignment of dental age or the assessment of dental development by looking into a child's mouth to note the teeth that have emerged through the gingiva. However, in the absence of other data, the number of teeth present are simply counted.[1]

When observations from clinical and radiographic sources of information are coupled with sufficient knowledge of dental morphology and the chronologies of the human dentition, the clinician has the foundation for the diagnosis and management of most disorders involving the size, shape, number, arrangement, esthetics, and development of the teeth and also problems related to the sequence of tooth eruption and occlusal relationships. For example, in Fig. 2.1A, the gingival tissues are excellent; however, the form of the maxillary incisors and interdental spacing might be considered to be an esthetic problem by a patient. To accept the patient's concern that a cosmetic problem is present and needs correction requires that the practitioner be able to transform the patient's idea of esthetics into reality by orthodontics and cosmetic

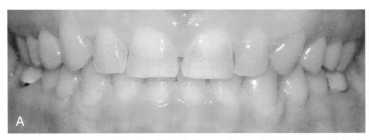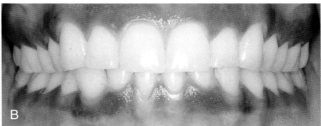

• **Fig. 2.1** Clinical observations: clinical crowns. Note the difference in the shapes of the teeth in (A) and (B), as well as the interdental spacing, and the presence and location of interproximal tooth contacts. Consider the contours of the roots (A), the occlusal contacts of the incisor, canine, and premolar teeth, and the gingiva of the maxillary right central incisor, and the esthetics presented in both (A) and (B). (A, From Ramfjord S, Ash MM: *Periodontology and periodontics,* Philadelphia, 1979, Saunders; B, From Ash MM: Paradigmatic shifts in occlusion and temporomandibular disorders, *J Oral Rehabil* 28:1–13, 2001.)

restorative dentistry. The situation in Fig. 2.1B demonstrates a periodontal problem (localized gingivitis of the gingival margin of the right central incisor), which is in part a result of the inadequate proximal contact relations of the incisors, leading to food impaction and accumulation of dental plaque and some calculus. However, for the most part, it is the result of inadequate home care hygiene. Most conservative correction relates to removal of the irritants and daily tooth brushing and dental flossing, especially of the interproximal areas of the central incisors. Even so, the risk factor of the inadequate proximal contact remains. If the form of a tooth is not consistent with its functions in the dental arches, it is highly probable that nonfunctional positions of interproximal contacts will lead to the problems indicated in Fig. 2.1B.

The form of every tooth is related to its position and angulation in the dental arch, its contact relations with the teeth in the opposing arch, its proximal contacts with adjacent teeth, and its relationship to the periodontium. An appreciation for the esthetics of tooth form and coloration is a requirement for the successful practitioner.

Variability

It is not enough to know just the "normal" morphology of the teeth; it is also necessary to accept the concept of morphologic variability in a functional, esthetic, and statistical sense. Most of the data on tooth morphology are derived from studies of samples of population of European-American ancestry (EAa), and, for example, as indicated in the section on Tooth Formation Standards in this chapter, a variety of sequences in eruption of the teeth exist depending on the population sampled. Because of the Immigration Reform Act of 1965, it is most likely that future tooth morphology standards will reflect the significant change in the ethnic makeup of the population of the United States (i.e., population samples of dentitions will reflect a greater variance).

Uncommon variations in the maxillary central incisors, which are shown in Chapter 6 (see Fig. 6.12), reflect samples drawn from a population made up largely of EAa. It is possible to accept the incisors shown as being representative of this population or perhaps "normal" for the EAa population at the time sampled. A shovel-shaped incisor trait is found in a Caucasoid population only infrequently (fewer than 5%); however, it is one of the characteristics found in patients with Down syndrome (trisomy 21) and normally in Chinese and Japanese individuals, Mongolians, and Eskimos. Statistically then, the shovel-shaped trait might be considered to be abnormal in the Caucasoid population but not so

in the Mongoloid populations. The practitioner must be prepared to adjust to such morphologic variations.

Malformations

It is necessary to know the chronologies of the primary and permanent dentitions to answer questions about when disturbances in the form, color, arrangement, and structure of the teeth might have occurred. Dental anomalies are seen most often with third molars, maxillary lateral incisors, and mandibular second premolars. Abnormally shaped crowns such as peg laterals and mandibular second premolars with two lingual cusps present restorative and space problems, respectively.

Patients who have a disturbance such as the ones shown in Fig. 2.2 not only want to know what to do about it, but they also want to know when or how the problem might have happened. How the problem came about is the most difficult part of the question. **Enamel hypoplasia** is a general term referring to all quantitative defects of enamel thickness. They range from single or multiple pits to small furrows and wide troughs to entirely missing enamel. Hypocalcification and opacities are qualitative defects. The location of defects on tooth crowns provides basic evidence for estimating the time of the development of the defect with an unknown error and potential bias.[2–5] One method of estimating is provided in the section Tooth Formation Standards.

In a cleft palate and lip, various associated malformations of the crowns of the teeth of both dentitions occur. The coronal malformations are not limited to the region of the cleft but involve posterior teeth as well.[6] A number of congenital malformations involving the teeth are evident, with some the result of endogenous factors and others the result of exogenous agents. When a malformation has some particular characteristics (e.g., screwdriver-shaped central incisors) and is consistent with a particular phase of dental development, it may be possible to determine the cause of the disturbance. This aspect is considered further in the section Dental Age.

Chronology of Primary Dentition

The chronology of the primary teeth presented in Table 2.1 is based on data derived from Tables 2.3 and 2.4. (The chronology of permanent teeth is discussed in Table 2.2.) The Universal numbering system is used in Table 2.1. The pictorial charts (Figs. 2.3 and 2.4) are not intended to be used as ideal standards of normal development. Their use is directed toward showing patients the general aspects of development rather than providing precise guidance for clinical procedures.

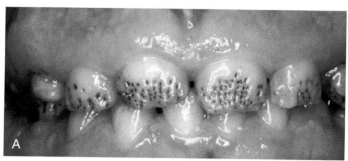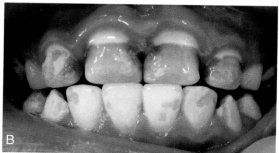

• **Fig. 2.2** (A) Hypoplasia of the enamel. (B) Defects in tooth structure caused by systemic fluorosis during development of the permanent dentition. (A, From Neville BW, Damm DD, Allen CM, et al: *Oral and maxillofacial pathology,* ed 3, St. Louis, 2009, Saunders.)

TABLE 2.1	Chronology of Primary Teeth				
	TOOTH	First Evidence of Calcification (Weeks in Utero)	Crown Completed (Months)	Eruption (Mean Age) (Months)	Root Completed (Years)
Upper					
i1	E, F	14	1½	10	1½
i2	D, G	16	2½	11	2
c	C, H	17	9	19	3¼
m1	B, I	15	6	16	2½
m2	A, J	19	11	29	3

Maxillary Teeth
Right A B C D E│F G H I J Left
           T S R Q P│O N M L K
Mandibular Teeth

Lower					
i1	P, O	14	2½	8	1½
i2	Q, N	16	3	13	1½
c	R, M	17	9	20	3¼
m1	S, L	15½	5½	16	2½
m2	T, K	18	10	27	3

Universal numbering system for primary/deciduous dentition; see Chapter 1. See Tables 2.3 and 2.4 for a detailed presentation of the data.
c, Canine; *i1,* Central incisor; *i2,* lateral incisor; *m1,* first molar; *m2,* second molar.

Development and Eruption/Emergence of the Teeth

Historically, the term *eruption* was used to denote the tooth's emergence through the gingiva, but then it became more completely defined to mean continuous tooth movement from the dental bud to occlusal contact.[7] However, not all tables of dental chronologies reflect the latter definition of eruption; the terms **eruption** and **emergence** are used here at this time in such a way as to avoid any confusion between the historical use of *eruption* and its more recent expanded meaning.

Emergence of the primary dentition takes place between the 6th and 30th months of postnatal life. It takes from 2 to 3 years for the primary dentition to be completed, beginning with the initial calcification of the primary central incisor to the completion of the roots of the primary second molar (see Fig. 2.3).

The emergence of the primary dentition through the alveolar mucous membrane is an important time for the development of oral motor behavior and the acquisition of masticator skills.[8] At this time of development, the presence of "teething" problems suggests how the primary dentition can affect the development of future neurobehavioral mechanisms, including jaw movements

TABLE 2.2   Chronology of Permanent Teeth

TOOTH		First Evidence of Calcification	Crown Completed (Years)	Emergence (Eruption) (Years)	Root Completed (Years)
I1	8, 9	3–4 months	4–5	7–8	10
I2	7, 10	10–12 months	4–5	8–9	11
C	6, 11	4–5 months	6–7	11–12	13–15
P1	5, 12	1½–1¾ years	5–6	10–11	12–13
P2	4, 13	2–2¼ years	6–7	10–12	12–14
M1	3, 14	At birth	2½–3	6–7	9–10
M2	2, 15	2½–3 years	7–8	12–13	14–16
M3	1, 16	7–9 years	12–16	17–21	18–25

Maxillary Teeth

Right 1   2   3   4   5   6   7   8 | 9   10   11   12   13   14   15   16 Left
     32 31 30 29 28 27 26 25 | 24 23 22 21 20 19 18 17

Mandibular Teeth

I1	24, 25	3–4 months	4–5	6–7	9
I2	23, 26	3–4 months	4–5	7–8	10
C	22, 27	4–5 months	6–7	9–10	12–14
P1	21, 28	1¼–2 years	5–6	10–12	12–13
P2	20, 29	2¼–2½ years	6–7	11–12	13–14
M1	19, 30	At birth	2½–3	6–7	9–10
M2	18, 31	2½–3 years	7–8	11–13	14–15
M3	17, 32	8–10 years	12–16	17–21	18–25

See Tables 2.3 and 2.4 in for a detailed presentation of the data.

C, Canine; *I1,* central incisor; *I2,* lateral incisor; *M1,* first molar; *M2,* second molar; *M3,* third molar; *P1,* first premolar; *P2,* second premolar.

and mastication. Learning of mastication may be highly dependent on the stage and development of the dentition (e.g., type and number of teeth present and occlusal relations), the maturation of the neuromuscular system, and such factors as diet.

Primary Teeth

Enamel organs (Fig. 2.5) do not all develop at the same rate; some teeth are completed before others are formed, which results in different times of eruption for different groups of teeth. Some of the primary/deciduous teeth are undergoing resorption while the roots of others are still forming. Not all the primary teeth are lost at the same time; some (e.g., central incisors) are lost 6 years before the primary canines. Groups of teeth develop at specific rates so that the sequence of eruption and emergence of the primary/deciduous teeth is well defined with few deviations. Even so, for the individual child, considerable variation in the times of emergence of the primary dentition may occur. The primary dentition is completely formed by approximately age 3 years and functions for a relatively short period before it is lost completely at approximately age 11. Permanent dentition is completed by approximately age 25 if the third molars are included (see Figs. 2.3 and 2.4).[9]

Calcification of the primary teeth begins in utero from 13 to 16 weeks postfertilization. By 18 to 20 weeks, all the primary teeth have begun to calcify. Primary tooth crown formation takes only approximately 2 to 3 years from initial calcification to root completion. However, mineralization of the permanent dentition is entirely postnatal, and the formation of each tooth takes approximately 8 to 12 years. The variability in tooth development is similar to that for eruption, sexual maturity, and other similar growth indicators.[10]

Crown formation of the primary teeth continues after birth for approximately 3 months for the central incisor, approximately 4 months for the lateral incisor, approximately 7 months for the primary first molar, approximately 8.5 months for the canine, and approximately 10.5 months for the second primary molar. During these periods before and after birth, disorders in shape, pigmentation, mineralization, and structure sometimes occur (fluorosis is considered later in this chapter).

Crown and Root Development

Dental development can be considered to have two components: (1) the formation of crowns and roots and (2) the eruption of the teeth. Of these two, the former seems to be much more resistant to environmental influences; the latter can be affected by caries and tooth loss.[11,12]

After the **crown** of the tooth is formed, development of the **root portion** begins. At the cervical border of the enamel (the cervix of the crown), cementum starts to form as a root covering of

TABLE 2.3	**Chronology of Human Dentition**				

Dentition	Tooth	FIRST EVIDENCE OF CALCIFICATION (Weeks in Utero)[a]	Crown Completed (Months)	Eruption (Months)[b,c]	Root Completed (Years)
Primary (upper)	i1	14 (13–16)	1½	10 (8–12)	1½
	i2	16 (14⅔–16½)[d]	2½	11 (9–13)	2
	c	17 (15–18)[d]	9	19 (16–22)	3¼
	m1	15½ (14½–17)	6	16 (13–19)♂ (14–18)♀	2½
	m2	19 (16–23½)	11	29 (25–33)	3
Primary (lower)	i1	14 (13–16)	2½	8 (6–10)	1½
	i2	16 (14⅔–)[d]	3	13 (10–16)	1½
	c	17 (16–)[d]	9	20 (17–23)	3¼
	m1	15½ (14½–17)	5½	16 (14–18)	2¼
	m2	18 (17–19½)	10	27 (23–31)♂ (24–30)♀	3
Permanent (upper)	I1	3–4 months	4–5 years	7–8 years	10
	I2	10–12 months	4–5 years	8–9 years	11
	C	4–5 months	6–7 years	11–12 years	13–15
	P1	1½–1¾ years	5–6 years	10–11 years	12–13
	P2	2–2¼ years	6–7 years	10–12 years	12–14
	M1	At birth	2½–3 years	6–7 years	9–10
	M2	2½–3 years	7–8 years	12–13 years	14–16
	M3	7–9 years	12–16 years	17–21 years	18–25
Permanent (lower)	I1	3–4 months	4–5 years	6–7 years	9
	I2	3–4 months	4–5 years	7–8 years	10
	C	4–5 months	6–7 years	9–10 years	12–14
	P1	1¾–2 years	5–6 years	10–12 years	12–13
	P2	2¼–2½ years	6–7 years	11–12 years	13–14
	M1	At birth	2½–3 years	6–7 years	9–10
	M2	2½–3 years	7–8 years	11–13 years	14–15
	M3	8–10 years	12–16 years	17–21 years	18–25

Part of the data from chronology of the growth of human teeth in Schour and Massler,[37] modified from Kronfeld[36] for permanent teeth, and Kronfeld and Schour[38] for the deciduous teeth. From Logan and Kronfeld,[39] slightly modified by McCall and Schour (in Orban[40]) and reflecting other chronologies:

[a]Kraus and Jordan[42];

[b]Lysell et al[13];

[c]mean age in months;

[d]Nomata[41]; Lunt and Law[19]; ±1 standard deviation; *c*, Canine; *i1*, central incisor; *i2*, lateral incisor; *m1*, first molar; *m2*, second molar; *M3*, third molar; *P1*, first premolar; *P2*, second premolar.

the dentin. The **cementum** is similar in some ways to bone tissue and covers the root of the tooth in a thin layer. In the absence of a succeeding permanent tooth, the root of the primary tooth may only partially resorb. When root resorption does not follow the usual pattern, the permanent tooth cannot emerge or is otherwise kept out of its normal place. In addition, the failure of the root to resorb may bring about prolonged retention of the primary tooth. Although mandibular teeth do not begin to move occlusally until crown formation is complete, their eruption rate does not closely correlate with root elongation. After the crown and part of the root are formed, the tooth penetrates the alveolar gingiva and makes its entry (emergence) into the mouth.

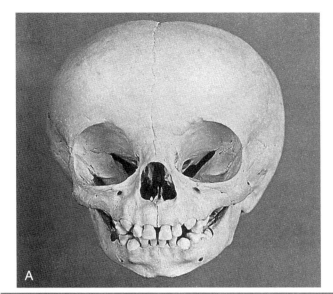

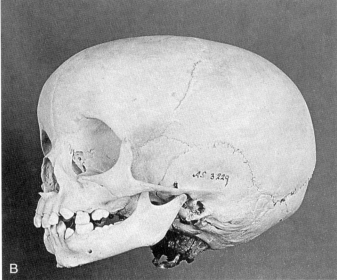

• **Fig. 2.7** Skull of a child approximately 20 months of age. (A) View showing all incisors present and erupting canines. (B) Lateral view. First primary molars are in occlusion; mandibular second molars are just emerging opposite the already erupted maxillary molar. (Modified from Karl W: *Atlas der Zahnheilkunde,* Berlin, [no publication date available], Verlag von Julius Springer.)

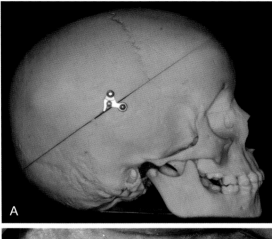

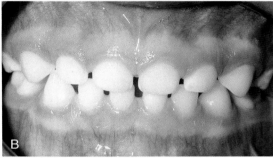

• **Fig. 2.8** (A), Skull of child 4 years old with completed primary dentition. (B) Completed primary dentition. Note the incisal wear. (A, Courtesy BoneClones, Osteological Reproductions. B, From Bird DL, Robinson DS: *Modern dental assisting,* ed 9, St. Louis, 2009, Saunders.)

Primary Dentition

The primary/deciduous dentition is considered to be completed by approximately 30 months or when the second primary molars are in occlusion (Fig. 2.8). The dentition period includes the time when no apparent changes occur intraorally (i.e., from approximately 30 months to approximately 6 years of age).

The form of the dental arch remains relatively constant without significant changes in depth or width. A slight increase in the intercanine width occurs about the time the primary incisors are lost, and an increase in size in both jaws in a sagittal direction is consistent with the space needed to accommodate the succedaneous teeth. An increase in the vertical dimension of the facial skeleton occurs as a result of alveolar bone deposition,

condyle growth, and deposition of bone at the synchondrosis of the basal part of the occipital bone and sphenoid bones, and at the maxillary suture complex.[20] The splanchnocranium remains small in comparison with the neurocranium. The part of the jaws that contain the primary teeth has almost reached adult width. At the first part of the transition period, which occurs at approximately age 8, the width of the mandible approximates the width of the neurocranium. The dental arches are complete, and the occlusion of the primary dentition is functional. During this period, attrition is sufficient in many children and is quite observable. The primary occlusion is considered in Chapter 16.

Transitional (Mixed) Dentition Period

The first transition dentition begins with the emergence and eruption of the permanent mandibular first molars and ends with the loss of the last primary tooth, which usually occurs at approximately age 11 to 12. The initial phase of the transition period lasts approximately 2 years, during which time the permanent first molars erupt (Figs. 2.9 and 2.10), the primary incisors are shed, and the permanent incisors emerge and erupt into position (Fig. 2.11). The permanent teeth do not begin eruptive movements until after the crown is completed. During eruption, the permanent mandibular first molar is guided by the distal surface of the second primary molar. If a distal step in the terminal plane is evident, malocclusion occurs (see Fig. 16.5).

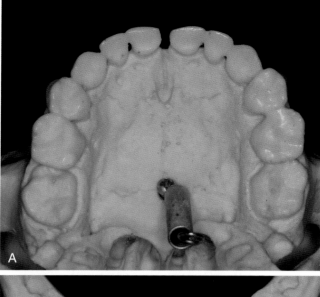

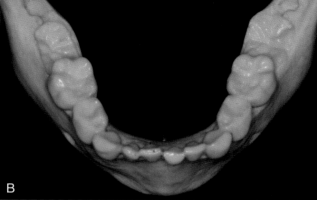

• **Fig. 2.9** Primary dentition with first permanent molars present. (A) Maxillary arch. (B) Mandibular arch. (Model courtesy BoneClones, Osteological Reproductions.)

Loss of Primary Teeth

The premature loss of primary teeth because of caries has an effect on the development of the permanent dentition.[21] This not only may reflect an unfortunate lack of knowledge as to the course of the disease but also establishes a negative attitude about preventing dental caries in the adult dentition. Loss of primary teeth may lead to the lack of space for the permanent dentition. It is sometimes assumed by laypersons that the loss of primary teeth, which are sometimes referred to as **baby teeth** or **milk teeth**, is of little consequence because they are only temporary. However, the primary dentition may be in use from age 2 to 7 or older, or approximately 5 or more years in all. Some of the teeth are in use from 6 months until 12 years of age, or 11.5 years in all. Thus these primary teeth are in use and contributing to the health and well-being of the individual during the first years of greatest development, physically and mentally.

Premature loss of primary teeth, retention of primary teeth, congenital absence of teeth, dental anomalies, and insufficient space are considered important factors in the initiation and development of an abnormal occlusion. Premature loss of primary teeth from dental neglect is likely to cause a loss of arch length with a consequent tendency for crowding of the permanent dentition. Arch length is considered in more detail in Chapter 16.

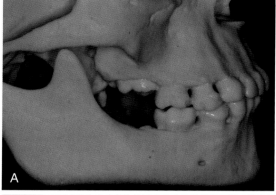

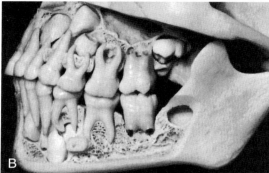

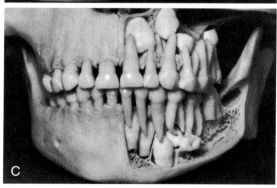

• **Fig. 2.10** Same child as in Fig. 2.9. (A) Right side. (B) Left side showing position of first permanent molars and empty bony crypt of developing second molar lost during preparation of the specimen. (C) Front view showing right side with bone covering roots and developing permanent teeth, and left side with developing anterior permanent teeth. (A, Model courtesy BoneClones, Osteological Reproductions.)

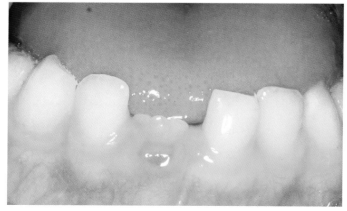

• **Fig. 2.11** Eruption of the permanent central incisor. Note the incisal edges demonstrating mamelons and the width of the emerging incisors.

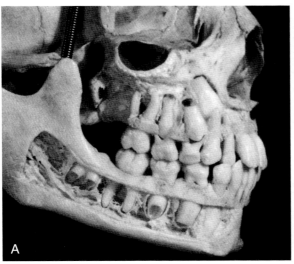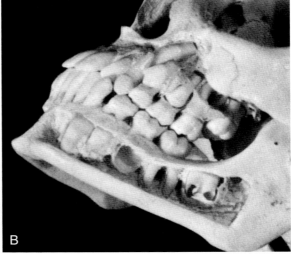

• **Fig. 2.12** (A) View of the right side of the skull of a child of 9 to 10 years of age. Note the amount of resorption of the roots of the primary maxillary molars, the relationship of the developing premolars above them, and the open pulp chambers and the pulp canals in the developing mandibular teeth. The roots of the first permanent molars have been completed. (B) Left side. Note the placement of the permanent maxillary canine and second premolar and the position and stage of development of the maxillary second permanent molar. The bony crypt of the lost mandibular second permanent premolar is in full view. Note the large openings in the roots of the mandibular second permanent molar.

Permanent Dentition

The permanent dentition consisting of 32 teeth is completed from 18 to 25 years of age if the third molar is included.

Apparently there are four or more **centers of formation** (developmental lobes) for each tooth. The formation of each center proceeds until a coalescence of all of them takes place. During this period of odontogenesis, injury to the developing tooth can lead to anomalous morphologic features (e.g., peg-shaped lateral incisor). Although no lines of demarcation are found in the dentin to show this development, signs are found on the surfaces of the crowns and roots; these are called **developmental grooves** (see Fig. 4.12B). Fractures of the teeth occur most commonly along these grooves (see Fig. 13.26).

The **follicles** of the developing **incisors** and **canines** are in a position lingual to the deciduous roots (see Fig. 2.10; see also Fig. 3.4).

The developing **premolars**, which eventually take the place of deciduous molars, are within the bifurcation of primary molar roots (Fig. 2.12A and B). The permanent incisors, canines, and premolars are called **succedaneous** teeth because they take the place of their primary predecessors.

The central incisor is the second permanent tooth to emerge into the oral cavity. Eruption time is quite close to that of the first molar (i.e., tooth emergence occurs between 6 and 7 years) (see Table 2.2). As with the first molar, at age 6 years, 50% of individuals have reached the stage considered to be the age of attainment of the stage or, more specifically, the age of emergence for the central incisor. The mandibular permanent teeth tend to erupt before maxillary teeth. The mandibular central incisor usually erupts before the maxillary central incisor (see Fig. 2.11) and may erupt simultaneously with or even before the mandibular first molar. The mandibular lateral incisor may erupt along with the central incisor.

Before the permanent central incisor can come into position, the primary central incisor must be exfoliated. This occurs through the resorption of the deciduous roots. The permanent tooth in its follicle attempts to move into the position held by its predecessor. Its influence on the primary root evidently causes resorption of the root, which continues until the primary crown has lost its anchorage, becomes loose, and is finally exfoliated. In the meantime, the permanent tooth has moved occlusally so that when the primary tooth is lost, the permanent one is at the point of eruption and in proper position to succeed its predecessor.

Mandibular lateral incisors erupt very soon after the central incisors, often simultaneously. The **maxillary central incisors** erupt next in chronologic order, and **maxillary lateral incisors** make their appearance approximately 1 year later (see Table 2.2 and Figs. 2.3 and 2.4). The **first premolars** follow the maxillary laterals in sequence when the child is approximately 10 years old; the **mandibular canines** (cuspids) often appear at the same time. The **second premolars** follow during the next year, and then the **maxillary canines** follow. Usually, the second molars come in when the individual is approximately 12 years of age; they are posterior to the first molars and are commonly called **12-year molars**.

The maxillary canines occasionally erupt along with the second molars, but in most instances of normal eruption, the canines precede them somewhat.

The **third molars** do not come in until age 17 or later. Considerable posterior jaw growth is required after age 12 to allow room for these teeth (Fig. 2.13). Third molars are subject to many anomalies and variations of form. Insufficient jaw development for their accommodation complicates matters in the majority of cases. Individuals who have properly developed third molars in good alignment are very much in the minority. Third-molar anomalies and variations with the complications brought about by misalignment and subnormal jaw development comprise a subject too vast to be covered here. Fig. 2.14 shows an anatomic specimen with a full complement of 32 teeth.

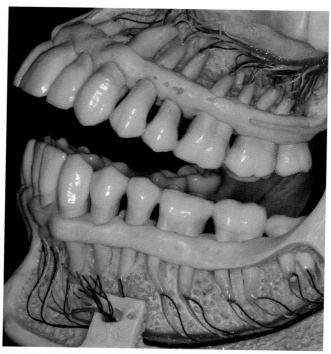

• **Fig. 2.13** Development of the maxillary and mandibular third molars. (Model courtesy Marcus Sommer SOMSO Modelle GmbH.)

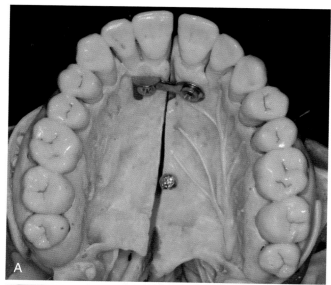

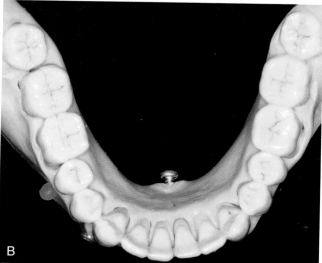

• **Fig. 2.14** Maxillary (A) and mandibular (B) arches with full complement of 32 teeth. (Model courtesy Marcus Sommer SOMSO Modelle GmbH.)

Size of Teeth

The size of teeth is largely genetically determined. However, marked racial differences do exist, as with the Lapps, a population with perhaps the smallest teeth, and the Australian aborigines, with perhaps the largest teeth.[22] Gender-size dimorphism differences average approximately 4% and are the greatest for the maxillary canine and the least for the incisors.[23] Often encountered is disharmony between the size of the teeth and bone size. Tooth size and arch size are considered in Chapter 16 relative to the development of occlusion.

Dental Pulp

The **dental pulp** is a connective tissue organ containing a number of structures, including arteries, veins, a lymphatic system, and nerves. Its primary function is to form the dentin of the tooth. When the tooth is newly erupted, the dental pulp is large; it becomes progressively smaller as the tooth is completed. The pulp is relatively large in primary teeth as well as in young permanent teeth (see Fig. 3.9). The teeth of children and young people are more sensitive than the teeth of older people to thermal change and dental operative procedures (heat generation). The opening of the pulp cavity at the apex is constricted and is called the **apical foramen**. The pulp keeps its tissue-forming function (e.g., to form **secondary dentin**), especially with the advance of dental caries toward the pulp. The pulp cavity becomes smaller and more constricted with age (see Fig. 13.3). The pulp chamber within the crown may become almost obliterated with a secondary deposit (e.g., osteodentin). This process is not as extensive in deciduous teeth.

Cementoenamel Junction

At the cementoenamel junction (CEJ) (see Figs. 1.3 and 1.4), visualized anatomically as the cervical line, the following several types of junctions are found: (1) the enamel overlapping the cementum, (2) an end-to-end approximating junction, (3) the absence of connecting enamel and cementum so that the dentin is an external part of the surface of the root, and (4) an overlapping of the enamel by the cementum. These different junctions have clinical significance in the presence of disease (e.g., gingivitis, recession of gingiva with exposure of CEJ, loss of attachment of supporting periodontal fibers in periodontitis); cervical sensitivity, caries, and erosion; and placement of the margins of dental restorations.

The CEJ is a significant landmark for probing the level of the attachment of fibers to the tooth in the presence of periodontal diseases. Using a periodontal probe (Fig. 2.15A), it is possible to relate the position of the gingival margin and the attachment to the CEJ (see Fig. 2.15B). Probing is done clinically to determine the level of periodontal support (regardless of whether a loss of

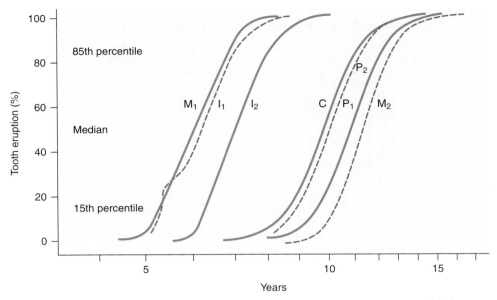

• **Fig. 2.20** Age of attainment of growth stage using a cumulative distribution function in which data represent tooth emergence. *C*, Canine; *I₁*, central incisor; *I₂*, lateral incisor; *M₁*, first molar; *M₂*, second molar; *P₁*, first premolar; *P₂*, second premolar. (Modified from Smith HB, Garn SM: Polymorphisms in eruption sequence of permanent teeth in American children, *Am J Phys Anthropol* 74:289–303, 1987.)

TABLE 2.7   Mean Age of Attainment of Developmental Stages for Females (Permanent Mandibular Teeth)

Developmental Stage	I1	I2	C	P1	P2	M1	M2	M3
C_i	—	—	0.5	1.8	3.0	0.0	3.5	9.6
C_{co}	—	—	0.8	2.2	3.6	0.3	3.7	10.1
C_{oc}	—	—	1.2	2.9	4.2	0.8	4.2	10.7
$Cr_{1/2}$	—	—	2.0	3.6	4.8	1.0	4.8	11.3
$Cr_{3/4}$	—	—	3.0	4.3	5.4	1.5	5.4	11.7
Cr_c	—	—	4.0	5.1	6.2	2.2	6.2	12.3
R_i	—	—	4.7	5.8	6.8	2.7	7.0	12.9
Cl_i	—	—	—	—	—	3.5	7.7	13.5
$R_{1/4}$	4.5	4.7	5.3	6.5	7.5	4.5	9.2	14.8
$R_{1/2}$	5.1	5.2	7.1	8.2	8.8	5.1	9.8	15.7
$R_{2/3}$	5.6	5.9	—	—	—	—	—	—
$2_{3/4}$	6.1	6.4	8.3	9.2	10.0	5.7	10.7	16.6
R_c	6.6	7.6	8.9	9.9	10.6	6.0	11.2	17.2
$A_{1/2}$	7.4	8.1	9.9	11.1	12.0	7.0	12.5	18.3
A_c	7.7	8.5	11.3	12.2	13.7	8.7	14.6	20.7

Values interpolated from Moorrees et al.[35]; all ages in years.[14]

$2_{3/4}$, Root three-fourths completed; $A_{1/2}$, apex half completed; A_c, apex completed; *C*, canine; C_{co}, cusp coalesced; C_i, Cusp initiated; Cl_i, initial cleft formation; C_{oc}, cusp outline completed; $Cr_{1/2}$, crown half completed; $Cr_{3/4}$, crown three-quarters completed; Cr_c, crown completed; *I1*, Central incisor; *I2*, lateral incisor; *M1*, first molar; *M2*, second molar; *M3*, third molar; *P1*, first premolar; *P2*, second premolar; $R_{1/2}$, root half completed; $R_{1/4}$, root one-fourth completed; $R_{2/3}$, root two-thirds completed; R_c, root completed; R_i, root initiated.

TABLE 2.8	Values for Predicting Age From Stages of Permanent Mandibular Tooth Formation—Females							
Developmental Stage	I1	I2	C	P1	P2	M1	M2	M3
C_i	—	—	0.6	2.0	3.3	0.2	3.6	9.9
C_{co}	—	—	1.0	2.5	3.9	0.5	4.0	10.4
C_{oc}	—	—	1.6	3.2	4.5	0.9	4.5	11.0
$Cr_{1/2}$	—	—	2.5	4.0	5.1	1.3	5.1	11.5
$Cr_{3/4}$	—	—	3.5	4.7	5.8	1.8	5.8	12.0
Cr_c	—	—	4.3	5.4	6.5	2.4	6.6	12.6
R_i	—	—	5.0	6.1	7.2	3.1	7.3	13.2
Cl_i	—	—	—	—	—	4.0	8.4	14.1
$R_{1/4}$	4.8	5.0	6.2	7.4	8.2	4.8	9.5	15.2
$R_{1/2}$	5.4	5.6	7.7	8.7	9.4	5.4	10.3	16.2
$R_{2/3}$	5.9	6.2	—	—	—	—	—	—
$R_{3/4}$	6.4	7.0	8.6	9.6	10.3	5.8	11.0	16.9
R_c	7.0	7.9	9.4	10.5	11.3	6.5	11.8	17.7
$A_{1/2}$	7.5	8.3	10.6	11.6	12.8	7.9	13.5	19.5
A_c	—	—	—	—	—	—	—	—

Values interpolated from Moorrees et al.[35]; all ages in years.[14]

See Table 2.7 for definitions of tooth designations and developmental stages.

$A_{1/2}$, apex half completed; A_c, apex completed; *C*, canine; C_{co}, cusp coalesced; C_i, Cusp initiated; Cl_i, initial cleft formation; C_{oc}, cusp outline completed; $Cr_{1/2}$, crown half completed; $Cr_{3/4}$, crown three-quarters completed; Cr_c, crown completed; *I1*, Central incisor; *I2*, lateral incisor; *M1*, first molar; *M2*, second molar; *M3*, third molar; *P1*, first premolar; *P2*, second premolar; $R_{1/2}$, root half completed; $R_{1/4}$, root one-fourth completed; $R_{2/3}$, root two-thirds completed; $R_{3/4}$, root three-fourths completed; R_c, root completed; R_i, root initiated.

Duration of Root and Crown Formation

The onset and duration of crown and root formation of the primary dentition are illustrated in Table 2.9, which answers questions about the relationship between onset and completion of tooth formation from start to finish.

Summary of Chronologies

Compared with older, descriptive chronologies based on dissection and those based on radiologic plus statistical methods to produce developmental data, newer methods tend to avoid attributing discrepancies to population differences because of methodologic or sampling effects. The data in Tables 2.7 and 2.8 have been recommended for deciduous tooth development.

Cumulative distribution functions and probit analysis are recommended for generating statistical solutions for schedules of age of attainment of growth stages.[14,35]

Clinicians can use chronologies to avoid treatment that can damage developing teeth (attainment schedules), to assess an unknown age of a patient (e.g., age prediction in forensics, demographics), and to assess growth (maturity).[14]

Sequence of Eruption

The sequence of eruption of the primary teeth does show some variation. Such timing is a result in large part of heredity and only somewhat of environmental factors. Jaw reversals in eruption of canines and first molars have been found to be important in increasing the variety of sequences.[13,60] When differences according to jaws are considered, Lunt and Law[19] conclude that the lateral incisor, first molar, and canine tend to erupt earlier in the maxilla than in the mandible. Sato and Ogiwara[60] found the following characteristic order in approximately one-third of their sample of children:

$$\frac{AB \quad D \quad C \quad E}{A \quad B \quad D \quad CE}$$

However, this arrangement of mean ages of eruption to yield a mean order of eruption was found to occur only in a small percentage of the participants in the study by Lysell et al.[13] The sequence and age of eruption of primary teeth are illustrated in Table 2.10.

Estimating Time of Enamel Hypoplasia

To estimate the time of enamel hypoplasia, measure in millimeters the distance from the CEJ to the midpoint of the enamel defect. As a comparison, note in Table 6.1 that the cervicoincisal length of the crown of the permanent maxillary central incisor is 10.5 mm. In Table 2.3 and Table 6.1, the first evidence of calcification is 3 to 4 months. Assuming that rate of development is constant and that a maxillary central incisor develops over 4 to 5 years, the age of development of the defect is related

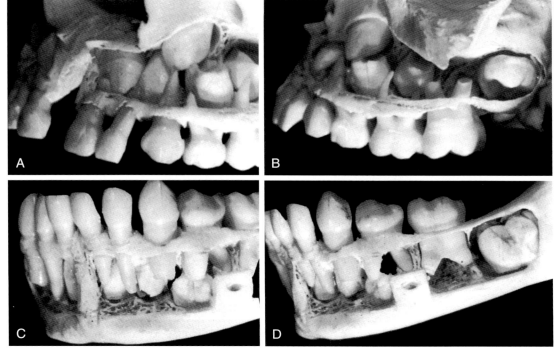

• **Fig. 3.5** A sectional close-up of the specimen in Fig. 3.4. (A) The left side of the maxilla. The developing crowns of the central and lateral incisors, the canine, and two premolars are clearly in view. (B) The left side of the maxilla, posteriorly. The molar relationship, both deciduous and permanent, is accented here. (C) This is a good view of the mandible anteriorly and to the left. Permanent central and lateral incisors and the canine may be seen. Notice that the permanent canine develops distally to the primary canine root. (D) Posteriorly, examination of the specimen mandible fails to find crown development of permanent premolars. However, the hollow spaces showing between the roots of primary molars may indicate a loss of material during the difficult process of dissection. The first permanent molar has progressed in crown formation, but the maturation of the whole tooth with alignment is far behind its opposition in the maxilla above it (see Fig. 3.4C).

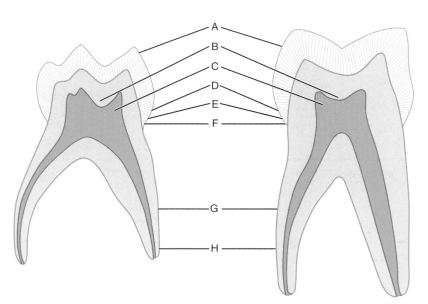

• **Fig. 3.6** Comparison of maxillary, primary, and permanent second molars, linguobuccal cross section. (A) The enamel cap of primary molars is thinner and has a more consistent depth. (B) A comparatively greater thickness of dentin is over the pulpal wall at the occlusal fossa of primary molars. (C) The pulpal horns are higher in primary molars, especially the mesial horns, and pulp chambers are proportionately larger. (D) The cervical ridges are more pronounced, especially on the buccal aspect of the first primary molars. (E) The enamel rods at the cervix slope occlusally instead of gingivally as in the permanent teeth. (F) The primary molars have a markedly constricted neck compared with the permanent molars. (G) The roots of the primary teeth are longer and more slender in comparison with crown size than those of the permanent teeth. (H) The roots of the primary molars flare out nearer the cervix than do those of the permanent teeth. (From Finn SB: *Clinical pedodontics,* ed 2, Philadelphia, 1957, Saunders.)

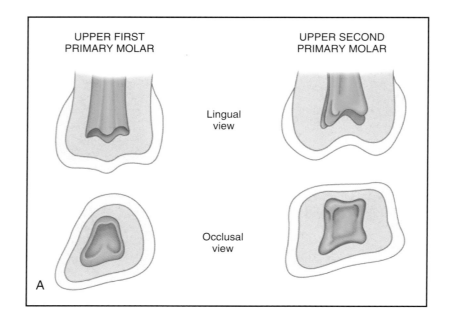

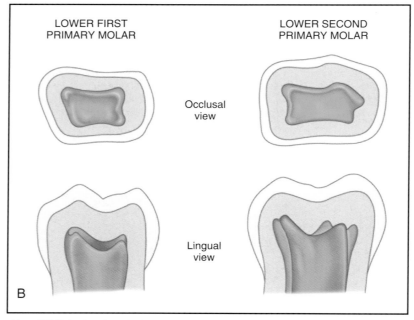

• **Fig. 3.7** (A and B) Pulp chambers in the primary molars. Note the contours of the pulp horns within them. (Modified from Finn SB: *Clinical pedodontics,* ed 2, Philadelphia, 1957, Saunders.)

2. The enamel is relatively thin and has a consistent depth.
3. The dentin thickness between the pulp chambers and the enamel is limited, particularly in some areas (lower second primary molar).
4. The pulp horns are high, and the pulp chambers are large (Fig. 3.7A and B).
5. Primary roots are narrow and long compared with crown width and length.
6. Molar roots of primary teeth flare markedly and thin out rapidly as the apices are approached.

Studying the comparisons between the deciduous and the permanent dentitions (Figs. 3.8 and 3.9) is of utmost importance. Discussion of further variations between the macroscopic form of the deciduous and the permanent teeth follows, with a detailed description of each deciduous tooth.

Detailed Description of Each Primary Tooth

Maxillary Central Incisor

Labial Aspect

In the crown of the primary central incisor, the mesiodistal diameter is greater than the cervicoincisal length (Figs. 3.10 and 3.11A). (The opposite is true of permanent central incisors.) The labial surface is very smooth, and the incisal edge is nearly straight. Developmental lines are usually not seen. The root is cone-shaped

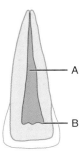

• **Fig. 3.8** Permanent central incisor. (A) Pulp canal; (B) pulp horns. This figure represents a sectioned central incisor of a young person. Although the pulp canal is rather large, it is smaller than the pulp canal shown in Fig. 3.9, and it becomes more constricted apically. Note the dentin space between the pulp horns and the incisal edge of the crown.

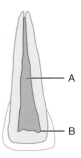

• **Fig. 3.9** Primary central incisor. (A) Pulp canal; (B) pulp horns. This figure represents a sectioned primary central incisor. The pulp chamber with its horns and the pulp canal are broader than those found in Fig. 3.8. The apical portion of the canal is much less constricted than that of the permanent tooth. Note the narrow dentin space incisally.

with even, tapered sides. The root length is greater in comparison with the crown length than that of the permanent central incisor. It is advisable when studying both the primary and permanent teeth to make direct comparisons between the table of measurements of the primary teeth (Table 3.1) and that of permanent teeth (see Table 1.1).

Lingual Aspect

The lingual aspect of the crown shows well-developed marginal ridges and a highly developed cingulum (Fig. 3.12A). The cingulum extends up toward the incisal ridge far enough to make a partial division of the concavity on the lingual surface below the incisal edge, practically dividing it into a mesial and distal fossa.

The root narrows lingually and presents a ridge for its full length in comparison with a flatter surface labially. A cross section through the root where it joins the crown shows an outline that is somewhat triangular in shape, with the labial surface making one side of the triangle and the mesial and distal surfaces the other two sides.

Mesial and Distal Aspects

The mesial and distal aspects of the primary maxillary central incisors are similar (Fig. 3.13A; see also Fig. 3.10). The measurement of the crown at the cervical third shows the crown from this aspect to be wide in relation to its total length. The average measurement is only about 1 mm less than the entire crown length cervicoincisally. Because of the short crown and its labiolingual measurement, the crown appears thick at the middle third and even down toward the incisal third. The **curvature of the cervical line**, which represents the **cementoenamel junction** (CEJ), is distinct, curving toward the incisal ridge. However, the curvature is not as great as that found on its

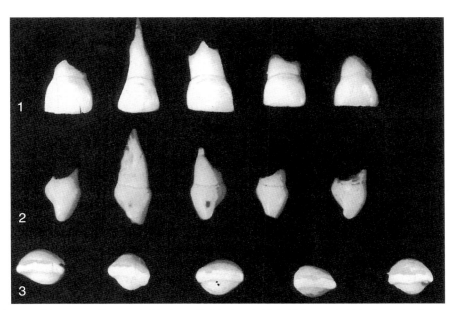

• **Fig. 3.10** Primary maxillary central incisors (first incisors). (1) Labial aspect. Note the lack of character in the mold form; also note the mesiodistal width compared with the shorter crown length. A little of the crown length was lost through abrasion before the date of extraction. (2) Mesial aspect. The cervical ridges are quite prominent labially and lingually, with the bulge much greater than that found on permanent incisors. This characteristic is common to each primary tooth to a varied degree. Normally, these curvatures are covered by gingival tissue with epithelial attachment (see Chapter 5). (3) Incisal aspect.

permanent successor. The cervical curvature distally is less than the curvature mesially, a design that compares favorably with the permanent central incisor.

Although the root appears blunter from this aspect than it did from the labial and lingual aspects, it is still of an even taper

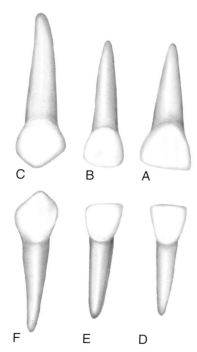

• **Fig. 3.11** Primary right anterior teeth, labial aspect. (A) Maxillary central incisor. (B) Maxillary lateral incisor. (C) Maxillary canine. (D) Mandibular central incisor. (E) Mandibular lateral incisor. (F), Mandibular canine.

and the shape of a long cone. However, it is blunt at the apex. Usually, the mesial surface of the root will have a developmental groove or concavity, whereas distally, the surface is generally convex.

Note the development of the cervical ridges of enamel at the cervical third of the crown labially and lingually.

Incisal Aspect

An important feature to note from the incisal aspect is the measurement mesiodistally compared with the measurement labiolingually (Fig. 3.14A; see also Fig. 3.10, 3). The incisal edge is centered over the main bulk of the crown and is relatively straight. Looking down on the incisal edge, the labial surface is much broader and also smoother than the lingual surface. The lingual surface tapers toward the cingulum.

The mesial and the distal surfaces of this tooth are relatively broad. The mesial and distal surfaces toward the incisal ridge or at the incisal third are generous enough to make good contact areas with the adjoining teeth, although this facility is used for a short period only because of rapid changes that take place in the jaws of children.

Maxillary Lateral Incisor

In general, the maxillary lateral is similar to the central incisor from all aspects, but its dimensions differ (Fig. 3.15; see also Figs. 3.11B, 3.12B, 3.13B, and 3.14B). Its crown is smaller in all directions. The cervicoincisal length of the lateral crown is greater than its mesiodistal width. The distoincisal angles of the crown are more rounded than those of the central incisor. Although the root has a similar shape, it is much longer in proportion to its crown than the central ratio indicates when a comparison is made.

TABLE 3.1 **Table of Measurements of the Primary Teeth of Man (Averages Only; in Millimeters)**

	Length Overall	Length of Crown	Length of Root	Mesiodistal Diameter of Crown	Mesiodistal Diameter of Crown at Cervix	Labiolingual Diameter of Crown	Labiolingual Diameter of Crown at Cervix
Upper Teeth							
Central incisor	16.0	6.0	10.0	6.5	4.5	5.0	4.0
Lateral incisor	15.8	5.6	11.4	5.1	3.7	4.0	3.7
Canine	19.0	6.5	13.5	7.0	5.1	7.0	5.5
First molar	15.2	5.1	10.0	7.3	5.2	8.5	6.9
Second molar	17.5	5.7	11.7	8.2	6.4	10.0	8.3
Lower Teeth							
Central incisor	14.0	5.0	9.0	4.2	3.0	4.0	3.5
Lateral incisor	15.0	5.2	10.0	4.1	3.0	4.0	3.5
Canine	17.5	6.0	11.5	5.0	3.7	4.8	4.0
First molar	15.8	6.0	9.8	7.7	6.5	7.0	5.3
Second molar	18.8	5.5	11.3	9.9	7.2	8.7	6.4

From Black GV: *Descriptive anatomy of the human teeth*, ed 4, Philadelphia, 1897, S.S. White Dental Company.

Maxillary Canine

Labial Aspect

Except for the root form, the labial aspect of the maxillary canine does not resemble either the central or the lateral incisor (Fig. 3.16; see also Fig. 3.11C). The crown is more constricted at the cervix in relation to its mesiodistal width, and the mesial and distal surfaces are more convex. Instead of an incisal edge that is relatively straight, it has a long, well-developed, sharp cusp.

Compared with that of the permanent maxillary canine, the cusp on the primary canine is much longer and sharper, and the crest of contour mesially is not as far down toward the incisal portion. A line drawn through the contact areas of the deciduous canine would bisect a line drawn from the cervix to the tip of the cusp. In the **permanent** canine, the contact areas are not at the same level. When the cusp is intact, the mesial slope of the cusp is longer than the distal slope. The root of the primary canine is long, slender, and tapering and is more than twice the crown length.

Lingual Aspect

The lingual aspect shows pronounced enamel ridges that merge with each other (see Fig. 3.12C). They are the cingulum, mesial, and distal marginal ridges and incisal cusp ridges, besides a tubercle at the cusp tip, which is a continuation of the lingual ridge connecting the cingulum and the cusp tip. This lingual ridge divides the lingual surface into shallow mesiolingual and distolingual fossae.

The root of this tooth tapers lingually. It is usually inclined distally also above the middle third (see Figs. 3.11C and 3.13C).

Mesial Aspect

From the mesial aspect, the outline form is similar to that of the lateral and central incisors (see Figs. 3.13C and 3.16, *2*). However, a difference in proportion is evident. The measurement labiolingually at the cervical third is much greater. This increase in crown dimension, in conjunction with the root width and length, permits resistance against forces the tooth must withstand during function. The function of this tooth is to punch, tear, and apprehend food material.

Distal Aspect

The distal outline of this tooth is the reverse of the mesial aspect. No outstanding differences may be noted, except that the curvature of the cervical line toward the cusp ridge is less than on the mesial surface.

Incisal Aspect

From the incisal aspect, we observe that the crown is essentially diamond-shaped (see Figs. 3.14C and 3.16, *3*). The angles that are found at the contact areas mesially and distally; the cingulum on the lingual surface; and the cervical third, or enamel ridge, on the labial surface are more pronounced and less rounded in effect than those found on the permanent canines. The tip of the cusp is distal to the center of the crown, and the mesial cusp slope is longer than the distal cusp slope. This allows for intercuspation with the lower, or mandibular, canine, which has its longest slope distally (see Fig. 3.11).

Mandibular Central Incisor

Labial Aspect

The labial aspect of this crown has a flat face with no developmental grooves (Fig. 3.17; see Fig. 3.11D). The mesial and distal sides of the crown are tapered evenly from the contact areas, with the measurement being less at the cervix. This crown is wide in

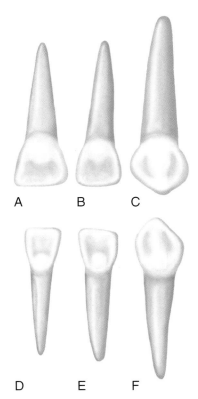

• **Fig. 3.12** Primary right anterior teeth, lingual aspect. (A) Maxillary central incisor. (B) Maxillary lateral incisor. (C) Maxillary canine. (D) Mandibular central incisor. (E) Mandibular lateral incisor. (F) Mandibular canine.

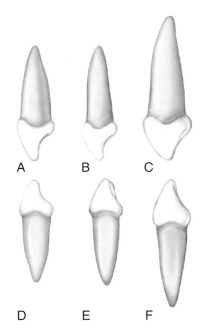

• **Fig. 3.13** Primary right anterior teeth, mesial aspect. (A) Maxillary central incisor. (B) Maxillary lateral incisor. (C) Maxillary canine. (D) Mandibular central incisor. (E) Mandibular lateral incisor. (F), Mandibular canine.

proportion to its length compared with that of its permanent successor. The heavy look at the root trunk makes this small tooth resemble the permanent maxillary lateral incisor.

The root of the primary central incisor is long and evenly tapered down to the apex, which is pointed. The root is almost twice the length of the crown (see Fig. 3.11D).

Lingual Aspect

On the lingual surface of the crown, the marginal ridges and the cingulum may be located easily (see Fig. 3.12D). The lingual surface of the crown at the middle third and the incisal third may have a flattened surface level with the marginal ridges, or it may present a slight concavity, called the **lingual fossa**. The lingual portion of the crown and root converges so that it is narrower toward the lingual and not the labial surface.

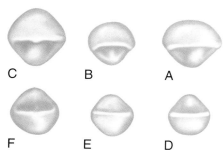

• **Fig. 3.14** Primary right anterior teeth, incisal aspect. (A) Maxillary central incisor. (B) Maxillary lateral incisor. (C) Maxillary canine. (D) Mandibular central incisor. (E) Mandibular lateral incisor. (F) Mandibular canine.

Mesial Aspect

The mesial aspect shows the typical outline of an incisor tooth, even though the measurements are small (see Figs. 3.13D and 3.17, *2*). The incisal ridge is centered over the center of the root and between the crest of curvature of the crown, labially, and lingually. The convexity of the cervical contours labially and lingually at the cervical third is just as pronounced as in any of the other primary incisors and more pronounced by far than the prominences found at the same locations on a permanent mandibular central incisor. As previously mentioned, these cervical bulges are important.

Although this tooth is small, its labiolingual measurement is only about a millimeter less than that of the primary maxillary central incisor. The primary incisors seem to be built for strenuous service.

The mesial surface of the root is almost flat and evenly tapered; the apex presents a more blunt appearance than found with the lingual or labial aspects.

Distal Aspect

The outline of this tooth from the distal aspect is the reverse of that found from the mesial aspect. Little difference can be noted between these aspects, except that the cervical line of the crown is less curved toward the incisal ridge than on the mesial surface. Often, a developmental depression is evident on the distal side of the root.

Incisal Aspect

The incisal ridge is straight and bisects the crown labiolingually. The outline of the crown from the incisal aspect emphasizes the

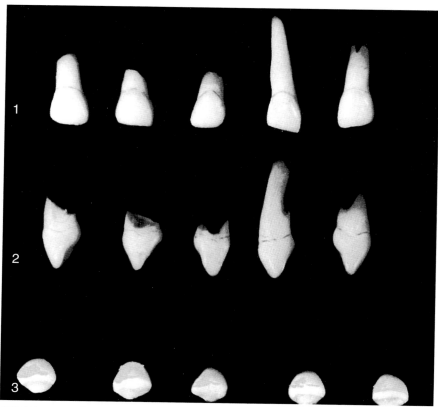

• **Fig. 3.15** Primary maxillary lateral incisors (second incisors). (1) Labial aspect. (2) Mesial aspect. (3) Incisal aspect.

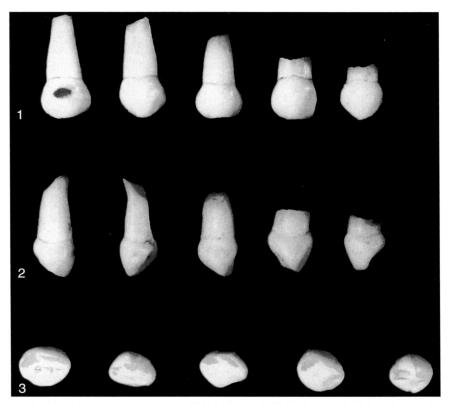

• **Fig. 3.16** Primary maxillary canines. (1) Labial aspect. (2) Mesial aspect. (3) Incisal aspect.

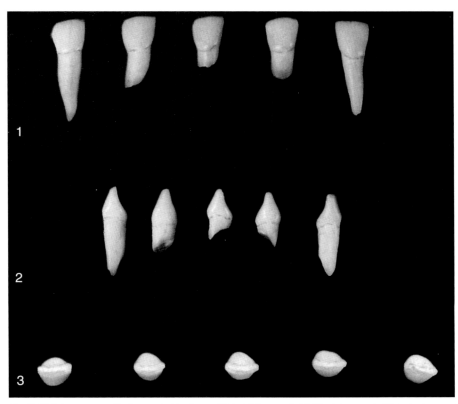

• **Fig. 3.17** Primary mandibular central incisors. (1) Labial aspect. (2) Mesial aspect. (3) Incisal aspect.

crests of contour at the cervical third labially and lingually (see Figs. 3.14D and 3.17, *3*). A definite taper is evident toward the cingulum on the lingual side.

The labial surface from this view presents a flat surface that is slightly convex, whereas the lingual surface presents a flattened surface that is slightly concave.

Mandibular Lateral Incisor

The fundamental outlines of the primary mandibular lateral incisor (Fig. 3.18) are similar to those of the primary central incisor. These two teeth supplement each other in function. The lateral incisor is somewhat larger in all measurements except labiolingually, where the two teeth are practically identical. The cingulum of the lateral incisor may be a little more generous than that of the central incisor. The lingual surface of the crown between the marginal ridges may be more concave. In addition, a tendency exists for the incisal ridge to slope downward distally. This design lowers the distal contact area apically, so that proper contact may be made with the mesial surface of the primary mandibular canine (see Figs. 3.11E, 3.12E, 3.13E, and 3.14E).

Mandibular Canine

Little difference in functional form is evident between the mandibular canine and the maxillary canine. The difference is mainly in the dimensions. The crown is perhaps 0.5 mm shorter, and the root is at least 2 mm shorter; the mesiodistal measurement of the mandibular canine at the root trunk is greater when compared with its mesiodistal measurement at the contact areas than is that of the maxillary canine (Fig. 3.19). It is "thicker" accordingly at the "neck" of the tooth. The outstanding variation in size between the two deciduous canines is shown by the labiolingual calibration. The deciduous maxillary canine is much larger labiolingually (see Fig. 3.13).

The cervical ridges labially and lingually are not quite as pronounced as those found on the maxillary canine. The greatest variation in outline form when one compares the two teeth is seen from the labial and lingual aspects; the distal cusp slope is longer than the mesial slope. The opposite arrangement is true of the maxillary canine. This makes for proper intercuspation of these teeth during mastication.

Fig. 3.20 illustrates the primary mandibular canines (see also Figs. 3.11F, 3.12F, 3.13F, and 3.14F).

Maxillary First Molar

Buccal Aspect

The widest measurement of the crown of the maxillary first molar is at the contact areas mesially and distally (Fig. 3.21A). From these points, the crown converges toward the cervix, with the measurement at the cervix being fully 2 mm less than the measurement at the contact areas. This dimensional arrangement furnishes a narrower look to the cervical portion of the crown and root of the primary maxillary first molar than that of the same portion of the permanent maxillary first molar. The occlusal line is slightly scalloped but with no definite cusp form. The buccal surface is smooth, and little evidence of developmental grooves is noted. It is from this aspect that one may judge the relative size of the primary maxillary first molar when it is compared with the second

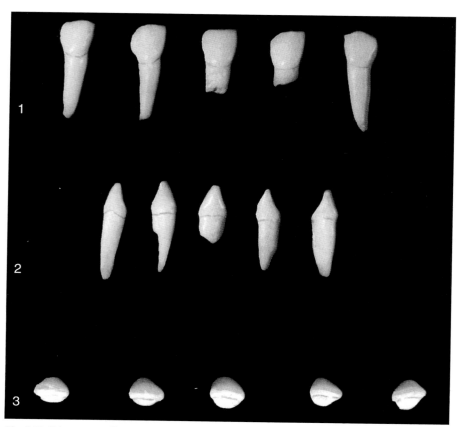

• **Fig. 3.18** Primary mandibular lateral incisors. (1) Labial aspect. (2) Mesial aspect. (3) Incisal aspect.

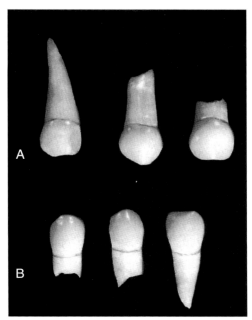

• **Fig. 3.19** A comparison of primary canines, both in the size and shape of the crowns. Two of them have their roots intact and show no dissolution. (A) Maxillary canines. (B) Mandibular canines. Compare Figs. 3.16 and 3.20.

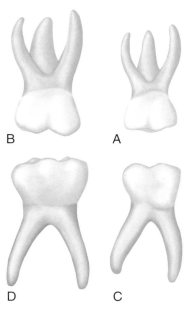

• **Fig. 3.21** Primary right molars, buccal aspect. (A) Maxillary first molar. (B) Maxillary second molar. (C) Mandibular first molar. (D) Mandibular second molar.

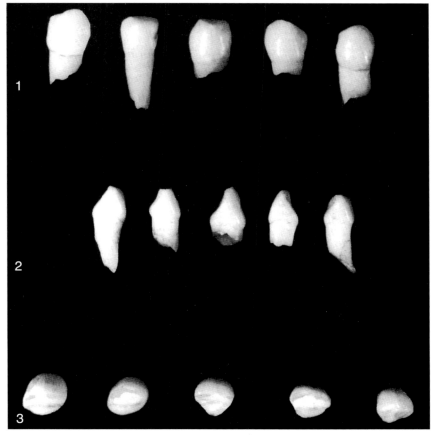

• **Fig. 3.20** Primary mandibular canines. (1) Labial aspect. (2) Mesial aspect. (3) Incisal aspect.

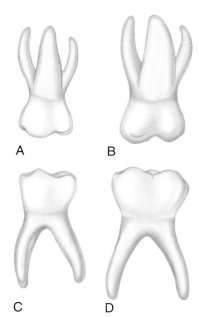

• **Fig. 3.22** Primary right molars, lingual aspect. (A) Maxillary first molar. (B) Maxillary second molar. (C) Mandibular first molar. (D) Mandibular second molar.

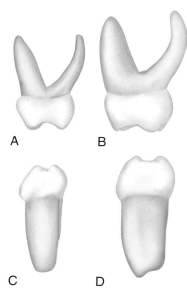

• **Fig. 3.23** Primary right molars, mesial aspect. (A) Maxillary first molar. (B) Maxillary second molar. (C) Mandibular first molar. (D), Mandibular second molar.

molar. It is much smaller in all measurements than the second molar. Its relative shape and size suggest that it was designed to be the "premolar section" of the primary dentition. In function it acts as a compromise between the size and shape of the anterior primary teeth and the molar area, this area being held temporarily by the larger primary second molar. At age 6 years, the large first permanent molar is expected to take its place distal to the second primary molar, which will complete a more extensive molar area for masticating efficiency.

The **roots** of the maxillary first molar are slender and long, and they spread widely. All three roots may be seen from this aspect. The distal root is considerably shorter than the mesial one. The bifurcation of the roots begins almost immediately at the site of the cervical line (CEJ). Actually, this arrangement is in effect for the entire root trunk, which includes a **trifurcation**, and this is a characteristic of all primary molars, whether maxillary or mandibular. Permanent molars do not possess this characteristic. The root trunk on permanent molars is much heavier, with a greater distance between the cervical lines to the points of bifurcations (see Fig. 11.8).

Lingual Aspect

The general outline of the lingual aspect of the crown is similar to that of the buccal aspect (Fig. 3.22A). The crown converges considerably in a lingual direction, which makes the lingual portion calibrate less mesiodistally than the buccal portion.

The mesiolingual cusp is the most prominent cusp on this tooth. It is the longest and sharpest cusp. The distolingual cusp is poorly defined; it is small and rounded when it exists at all. From the lingual aspect, the distobuccal cusp may be seen, since it is longer and better developed than the distolingual cusp. A type of primary maxillary first molar that is not uncommon and presents as one large lingual cusp with no developmental groove in evidence lingually is a three-cusped molar (see Fig. 3.25, *4*, second from left).

All three roots also may be seen from this aspect. The lingual root is larger than the others.

Mesial Aspect

From the mesial aspect, the dimension at the cervical third is greater than the dimension at the occlusal third (Fig. 3.23A). This is true of all molar forms, but it is more pronounced on primary than on permanent teeth. The mesiolingual cusp is longer and sharper than the mesiobuccal cusp. A pronounced convexity is evident on the buccal outline of the cervical third. This convexity is an outstanding characteristic of this tooth. It actually gives the impression of overdevelopment in this area when comparisons are made with any other tooth, primary or permanent, with the mandibular first primary molar being a close contender. The cervical line mesially shows some curvature in the direction of the occlusal surface.

The mesiobuccal and lingual roots are visible only when looking at the mesial side of this tooth from a point directly opposite the contact area. The distobuccal root is hidden behind the mesiobuccal root. The lingual root from this aspect looks long and slender and extends lingually to a marked degree. It curves sharply in a buccal direction above the middle third.

Distal Aspect

From the distal aspect, the crown is narrower distally than mesially; it tapers markedly toward the distal end (Fig. 3.24A). The distobuccal cusp is long and sharp, and the distolingual cusp is poorly developed. The prominent bulge seen from the mesial aspect at the cervical third does not continue distally. The cervical line may curve occlusally, or it may extend straight across from the buccal surface to the lingual surface. All three roots may be seen from this angle, but the distobuccal root is superimposed on the mesiobuccal root so that only the buccal surface and the apex of the latter may be seen. The point of bifurcation of the distobuccal root and the lingual root is near the CEJ and, as described earlier, is typical.

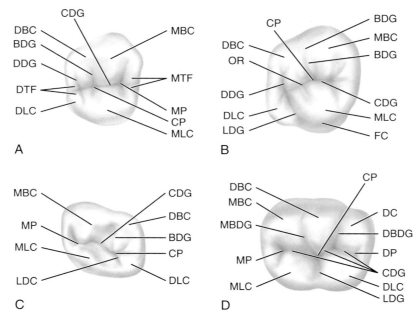

• **Fig. 3.24** (A) Maxillary first molar. *BDG,* Buccal developmental groove; *CDG,* central developmental groove; *CP,* central pit; *DBC,* distobuccal cusp; *DDG,* distal developmental groove; *DLC,* distolingual cusp; *DTF,* distal triangular fossa; *MBC,* Mesiobuccal cusp; *MLC,* mesiolingual cusp; *MP,* mesial pit; *MTF,* mesial triangular fossa. (B) Maxillary second molar. *BDG,* Buccal developmental groove; *CDG,* central developmental groove; *CP,* central pit; *DBC,* distobuccal cusp; *DDG,* distal developmental groove; *DLC,* distolingual cusp; *FC,* fifth cusp; *LDG,* lingual developmental groove; *MBC,* mesiobuccal cusp; *MLC,* mesiolingual cusp; *OR,* oblique ridge. (C) Mandibular first molar. *BDG,* Buccal developmental groove; *CDG,* Central developmental groove; *CP,* central pit; *DBC,* distobuccal cusp; *DLC,* distolingual cusp; *LDC,* lingual developmental groove; *MBC,* mesiobuccal cusp; *MLC,* mesiolingual cusp; *MP,* mesial pit. (D) Mandibular second molar. *CDG,* Central developmental groove; *CP,* central pit; *DBC,* Distobuccal cusp; *DBDG,* distobuccal developmental groove; *DC,* distal cusp; *DLC,* distolingual cusp; *DP,* distal pit; *LDG,* lingual developmental groove; *MBC,* mesiobuccal cusp; *MBDG,* mesiobuccal developmental groove; *MLC,* mesiolingual cusp; *MP,* mesial pit.

Occlusal Aspect

The calibration of the distance between the mesiobuccal line angle and the distobuccal line angle is definitely greater than the calibration between the mesiolingual line angle and the distolingual line angle (see Fig. 3.24A). Therefore the crown outline converges lingually. Also, the calibration from the mesiobuccal line angle to the mesiolingual line angle is definitely greater than that found at the distal line angles. Therefore the crown also converges distally. Nevertheless, these convergences are not reflected entirely in the working occlusal surface because it is more nearly rectangular, with the shortest sides of the rectangle represented by the marginal ridges. The occlusal surface has a **central fossa**. A **mesial triangular fossa** is just inside the mesial marginal ridge, with a mesial pit in this fossa and a sulcus with its central groove connecting the two fossae. A well-defined **buccal developmental groove** divides the mesiobuccal cusp and the distobuccal cusp occlusally. Supplemental grooves radiate from the pit in the mesial triangular fossa as follows: one buccally, one lingually, and one toward the marginal ridge, with the last sometimes extending over the marginal ridge mesially.

Sometimes the primary maxillary first molar has a well-defined triangular ridge connecting the mesiolingual cusp with the distobuccal cusp. When well developed, it is called the **oblique ridge**. In some of these teeth, the ridge is indefinite, and the central developmental groove extends from the mesial pit to the **distal developmental groove**. This disto-occlusal groove is always seen and may or may not extend through to the lingual surface, outlining a distolingual cusp. The distal marginal ridge is thin and poorly developed in comparison with the mesial marginal ridge.

Summary of the Occlusal Aspect of the Maxillary First Primary Molar

The form of the maxillary first primary molar varies from that of any tooth in the permanent dentition. Although no premolars are in the primary set, in some respects the crown of this primary molar resembles a permanent maxillary premolar. Nevertheless, the divisions of the occlusal surface and the root form with its efficient anchorage make it a molar, both in type and function. Fig. 3.25 presents all the aspects of the primary maxillary first molars.

Maxillary Second Molar

Buccal Aspect

The primary maxillary second molar has characteristics resembling those of the *permanent* maxillary first molar, but it is smaller (see Fig. 3.21B). The buccal view of this tooth shows two well-defined buccal cusps with a buccal developmental groove between them (Fig. 3.26, *1*). In line with all primary molars, the crown is narrow at the cervix in comparison with its mesiodistal measurement at the contact areas. This crown is much larger than that of the first primary molar. Although from this aspect

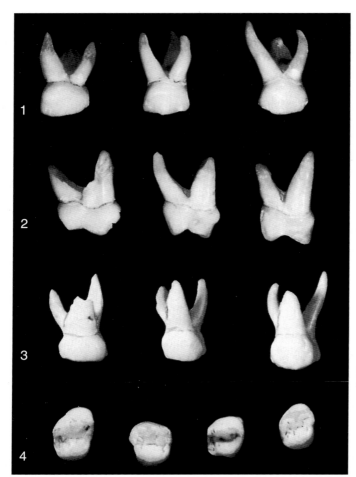

• **Fig. 3.25** Primary maxillary first molars. (1) Buccal aspect. Note the flare of roots. (2) Mesial aspect. The cervical ridge on the buccal surface is curved to the extreme. Also note the flat or concave buccal surface above this bulge as it approaches the occlusal surface. (3) Lingual aspect. (4) Occlusal aspect. This aspect emphasizes the extensive width of the mesial portion of primary first molars. The four specimens show size differentials even in deciduous teeth (see Fig. 3.24).

the roots appear slender, they are much longer and heavier than those that are a part of the maxillary first molar. The point of bifurcation between the buccal roots is close to the cervical line of the crown. The two buccal cusps are more nearly equal in size and development than those of the primary maxillary first molar.

Lingual Aspect

Lingually, the crown shows the following three cusps: (1) the mesiolingual cusp, which is large and well developed; (2) the distolingual cusp, which is well developed (more so than that of the primary first molar); and (3) a third supplemental cusp, which is apical to the mesiolingual cusp and sometimes called the **tubercle of Carabelli**, or the fifth cusp (see Fig. 3.22B). This cusp is poorly developed and merely acts as a buttress or supplement to the bulk of the mesiolingual cusp. If the tubercle of Carabelli seems to be missing, some traces of developmental lines or "dimples" remain (see Fig. 3.26, *3*). A well-defined developmental groove separates the mesiolingual cusp from the distolingual cusp and connects with the developmental groove, which outlines the fifth cusp.

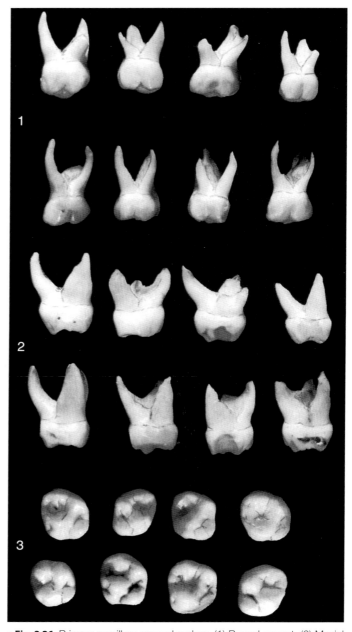

• **Fig. 3.26** Primary maxillary second molars. (1) Buccal aspect. (2) Mesial aspect. (3) Occlusal aspect.

All three roots are visible from this aspect; the lingual root is large and thick compared with the other two roots. It is approximately the same length as the mesiobuccal root. If it should differ, it will be on the short side.

Mesial Aspect

From the mesial aspect, the crown has a typical molar outline that greatly resembles that of the permanent molars (see Figs. 3.23B and 3.26, *2*). The crown appears short because of its width buccolingually in comparison with its length. The crown of this tooth is usually only about 0.5 mm longer than the crown of the first deciduous molar, but the buccolingual measurement is 1.5 to 2 mm greater. In addition, the roots are 1.5 to 2 mm longer. The mesiolingual cusp of the crown with its supplementary fifth cusp appears large in comparison with the mesiobuccal cusp. The mesiobuccal cusp from this angle is relatively short and sharp. Little curvature to the cervical line is evident. Usually, it is almost straight across from the buccal surface to lingual surface.

The mesiobuccal root from this aspect is broad and flat. The lingual root has somewhat the same curvature as the lingual root of the maxillary first deciduous molar.

The mesiobuccal root extends lingually far out beyond the crown outline. The point of bifurcation between the mesiobuccal root and the lingual root is 2 or 3 mm apical to the cervical line of the crown; this differs in depth on the root trunk from comparisons of this area in the recent discussion of primary molars. The mesiobuccal root presents itself as being quite wide from the mesial aspect. It measures approximately two-thirds the width of the root trunk, which leaves one-third for the lingual root. The mesiolingual cusp is directly below their bifurcation. Although from this aspect the curvature is strong lingually at the cervical portion, as on most deciduous teeth the crest of curvature buccally at the cervical third is nominal and resembles the curvature found at this point on the permanent maxillary first molar. In this, it differs entirely from the prominent curvature found on the primary maxillary first molars at the cervical third buccally.

Distal Aspect

From the distal aspect, it is apparent that the distal calibration of the crown is less than the mesial measurement, but the variation is found on the crown of the deciduous maxillary first molar. From both the distal and mesial aspects, the outline of the crown lingually creates a smooth, rounded line, whereas a line describing the buccal surface is almost straight from the crest of curvature to the tip of the buccal cusp. The distobuccal cusp and the distolingual cusp are about the same in length. The cervical line is approximately straight, as was found mesially.

All three roots are seen from this aspect, although only a part of the outline of the mesiobuccal root may be seen, because the distobuccal root is superimposed over it. The distobuccal root is shorter and narrower than the other roots. The point of bifurcation between the distobuccal root and the lingual root is more apical in location than any of the other points of bifurcation. The point of bifurcation between these two roots on the distal is more nearly centered above the crown than that on the mesial between the mesiobuccal and lingual roots.

Occlusal Aspect

From the occlusal aspect, this tooth resembles the permanent first molar (see Figs. 3.24 and 3.26, 3). It is somewhat rhomboidal and has four well-developed cusps and one supplemental cusp: mesiobuccal, distobuccal, mesiolingual, distolingual, and fifth cusps. The buccal surface is rather flat with the developmental groove between the cusps less marked than that found on the first permanent molar. Developmental grooves, pits, oblique ridge, and others are almost identical. The character of the "mold" is constant.

The occlusal surface has a *central fossa* with a **central pit**, a well-defined *mesial triangular fossa*, just distal to the **mesial marginal ridge**, with a mesial pit at its center. A well-defined developmental groove called the **central groove** is also at the bottom of a sulcus, connecting the mesial triangular fossa with the central fossa. The *buccal developmental groove* extends buccally from the central pit, separating the triangular ridges, which are occlusal continuations of the mesiobuccal and distobuccal cusps. Supplemental grooves often radiate from these developmental grooves.

The *oblique ridge* is prominent and connects the mesiolingual cusp with the distobuccal cusp. Distal to the oblique ridge,

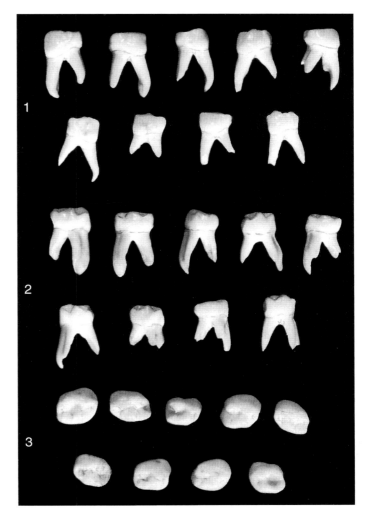

• **Fig. 3.27** Primary mandibular first molars. This tooth has characteristics unlike those of any other tooth in the mouth, primary or permanent. (1) Buccal aspect. (2) Lingual aspect. (3) Occlusal aspect.

the **distal fossa** is found, which harbors the *distal developmental groove*. The distal groove has branches of supplemental grooves within the **distal triangular fossa**, which is rather indefinitely outlined just mesial to the distal marginal ridge.

The distal groove acts as a line of demarcation between the mesiolingual and distolingual cusps and continues on to the lingual surface as the **lingual developmental groove**. The **distal marginal ridge** is as well developed as the *mesial marginal ridge*. It should be remembered that the marginal ridges are not developed equally on the primary maxillary first molar.

Mandibular First Molar

The mandibular first molar does not resemble any of the other teeth, deciduous or permanent. Because it varies so much from all others, it appears strange and primitive (Fig. 3.27).

Buccal Aspect

From the buccal aspect, the mesial outline of the crown of the primary mandibular first molar is almost straight from the contact area to the cervix, constricting the crown very little at the cervix (Fig. 3.28A). The outline describing the distal portion,

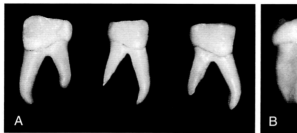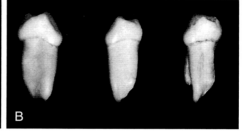

• **Fig. 3.28** Three rare specimens of the primary mandibular first molars. (A) Buccal aspect. (B) Mesial aspect. These three specimens have their roots intact with little or no resorption showing. They enable the viewer to observe the actual shape and size of the mesial and distal roots. The mesial root is broad, curved, and long, with fluting down the center. This makes for tremendous anchorage. The distal root is much shorter, but it is heavy and also curved. It does its share in bracing the crown, being in partnership with the mesial root during the process.

however, converges toward the cervix more than usual, so that the contact area extends distally to a marked degree (see Figs. 3.21C and 3.27, *1*).

The distal portion of the crown is shorter than the mesial portion, with the cervical line dipping apically where it joins the mesial root.

The two buccal cusps are rather distinct, although no developmental groove is evident between them. The mesial cusp is larger than the distal cusp. A developmental depression dividing them (not a groove) extends over to the buccal surface.

The roots are long and slender, and they spread greatly at the apical third beyond the outline of the crown.

The buccal aspect emphasizes the strange, primitive look of this tooth. The primary first mandibular molar from this angle impresses one with the thought of the possibility that at some time in the dim past, a fusion of two teeth ended in a strange single combination. That thought seems particularly apropos when a well-formed specimen of the tooth in question is located—one with its roots intact, showing no evidences of decalcification.

From the buccal aspect, if a line is drawn from the bifurcation of the roots to the occlusal surface, the tooth will be evenly divided mesiodistally. However, the mesial portion represents a tooth with a crown almost twice as tall as the distal half, and the root is again a third longer than the distal one. Two complete teeth are represented, but their dimensions differ considerably (see Figs. 3.21C and 3.27, *1*).

Lingual Aspect

The crown and root converge lingually to a marked degree on the mesial surface (see Figs. 3.22C and 3.27, *2*). Distally, the opposite arrangement is true of both crown and root. The distolingual cusp is rounded and suggests a developmental groove between this cusp and the mesiolingual cusp. The mesiolingual cusp is long and sharp at the tip, more so than any of the other cusps. The sharp and prominent mesiolingual cusp (almost centered lingually but in line with the mesial root) is an outstanding characteristic found occlusally on the primary first mandibular molar. It is noted that the mesial marginal ridge is so well developed that it might almost be considered another small cusp lingually. Part of the two buccal cusps may be seen from this angle.

From the lingual aspect, the crown length mesially and distally is more uniform than it is from the buccal aspect. The cervical line is straighter.

Mesial Aspect

The most noticeable detail from the mesial aspect is the extreme curvature buccally at the cervical third (see Fig. 3.28B). Except for this detail, the crown outline of this tooth from this aspect resembles the mesial aspect of the primary second molar and that aspect of the permanent mandibular molars. In this comparison, the buccal cusps are placed over the root base, and the lingual outline of the crown extends out lingually beyond the confines of the root base.

Both the mesiobuccal cusp and the mesiolingual cusp are in view from this aspect, as is the well-developed mesial marginal ridge. Because the mesiobuccal is greater than the mesiolingual crown length, the cervical line slants upward buccolingually. Note the flat appearance of the buccal outline of the crown from the crest of curvature of the buccal surface at the cervical third to the tip of the mesiobuccal cusp. All the primary molars have flattened buccal surfaces above this cervical ridge.

The outline of the mesial root from the mesial aspect does not resemble the outline of *any other primary tooth root*. The buccal and lingual outlines of the root drop straight down from the crown and are approximately parallel for more than half their length, tapering only slightly at the apical third. The root end is flat and almost square. A developmental depression usually extends almost the full length of the root on the mesial side.

Distal Aspect

The distal aspect of the mandibular first molar differs from the mesial aspect in several ways. The cervical line does not drop buccally. The length of crown buccally and lingually is more uniform, and the cervical line extends almost straight across buccolingually. The distobuccal cusp and the distolingual cusp are not as long or as sharp as the two mesial cusps. The distal marginal ridge is not as straight or well defined as the mesial marginal ridge. The distal root is rounder and shorter and tapers more apically.

Occlusal Aspect

The general outline of this tooth from the occlusal aspect is rhomboidal (see Fig. 3.27, *3*). The prominence present mesiobuccally is noticeable from this aspect, which accents the mesiobuccal line angle of the crown in comparison with the distobuccal line angle and thereby emphasizes the rhomboidal form.

The mesiolingual cusp may be seen as the largest and best developed of all the cusps, and it has a broad, flattened surface lingually. The buccal developmental groove of the occlusal surface

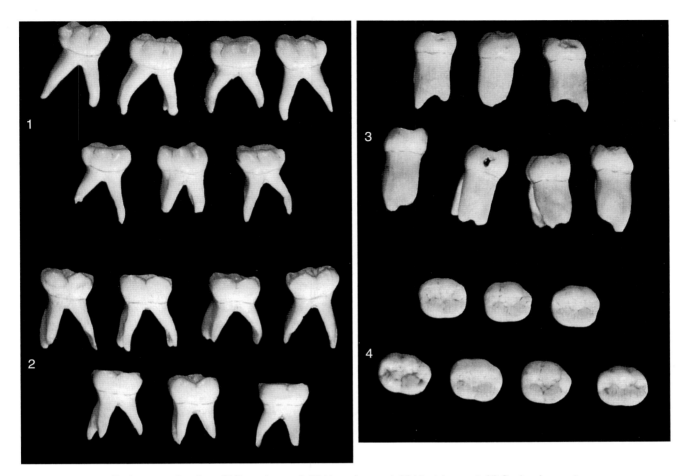

• **Fig. 3.29** Primary mandibular second molars. (1) Buccal aspect. (2) Lingual aspect. (3) Mesial aspect. (4) Occlusal aspect.

divides the two buccal cusps evenly. This developmental groove is short, extending from between the buccal cusp ridges to a point approximately in the center of the crown outline at a central pit. The central developmental groove joins it at this point and extends mesially, separating the mesiobuccal cusp and the mesiolingual cusp. The central groove ends in a mesial pit in the mesial triangular fossa, which is immediately distal to the mesial marginal ridge. Two supplemental grooves join the developmental groove in the center of the mesial triangular fossa; one supplemental groove extends buccally and the other extends lingually.

The mesiobuccal cusp exhibits a well-defined triangular ridge on the occlusal surface, which terminates in the center of the occlusal surface buccolingually at the *central developmental groove*. The *lingual developmental groove* extends lingually from this point, separating the mesiolingual cusp and the distolingual cusp. Usually, the lingual developmental groove does not extend through to the lingual surface but stops at the junction of lingual cusp ridges. Some supplemental grooves immediately mesial to the *distal marginal ridge* in the *distal triangular fossa* join with the central developmental groove.

Mandibular Second Molar

The primary mandibular *second* molar has characteristics that resemble those of the *permanent* mandibular *first* molar, although its dimensions differ (Fig. 3.29).

Buccal Aspect

From the buccal aspect, the primary mandibular second molar has a narrow mesiodistal calibration at the cervical portion of the crown compared with the calibration mesiodistally on the crown at contact level. The mandibular first permanent molar, accordingly, is wider at the cervical portion (see Figs. 3.21D, and 3.29, *1*).

From this aspect also, mesiobuccal and distobuccal developmental grooves divide the buccal surface of the crown occlusally into three cuspal portions almost equal in size. This arrangement forms a straight buccal surface presenting a mesiobuccal, a buccal, and a distobuccal cusp. It differs, therefore, from the mandibular **first permanent** molar, which has an uneven distribution buccally, presenting two buccal cusps and one distal cusp.

The roots of the primary second molar from this angle are slender and long. They have a characteristic flare mesiodistally at the middle and apical thirds. The roots of this tooth may be twice as long as the crown.

The point of bifurcation of the roots starts immediately below the CEJ of crown and root.

Lingual Aspect

From the lingual aspect, two cusps of almost equal dimensions can be observed (see Figs. 3.22D and 3.29, *2*). A short, lingual groove is between them. The two lingual cusps are not quite as wide as the three buccal cusps; this arrangement narrows the crown lingually. The cervical line is relatively straight, and the crown extends out over the root more distally than it does mesially. The mesial portion of the crown seems to be a little higher than the distal portion of the crown when viewed from the lingual aspect. It gives the impression of being tipped distally. A portion of each of the three buccal cusps may be seen from this aspect.

The roots from this aspect give somewhat the same appearance as from the buccal aspect. Note the length of the roots.

Mesial Aspect

From the mesial aspect, the outline of the crown resembles that of the permanent mandibular first molar (see Figs. 3.23D and 3.29, 3). The crest of contour buccally is more prominent on the primary molar, and the tooth seems to be more constricted occlusally because of the flattened buccal surface above this cervical ridge.

The crown is poised over the root of this tooth in the same manner as all mandibular posteriors; its buccal cusp is over the root and the lingual outline of the crown extending out beyond the root line. The marginal ridge is high, a characteristic that makes the mesiobuccal cusp and the mesiolingual cusp appear rather short. The lingual cusp is longer, or higher, than the buccal cusp. The cervical line is regular, although it extends upward buccolingually, making up for the difference in length between the buccal and lingual cusps.

The mesial root is unusually broad and flat with a blunt apex that is sometimes serrated.

Distal Aspect

The crown is not as wide distally as it is mesially; therefore it is possible to see the mesiobuccal and distobuccal cusps from the distal aspect. The distolingual cusp appears well developed, and the triangular ridge from the tip of this cusp extending down into the occlusal surface is seen over the distal marginal ridge.

The distal marginal ridge dips down more sharply and is shorter buccolingually than the mesial marginal ridge. The cervical line of the crown is regular, although it has the same upward incline buccolingually on the distal as on the mesial.

The distal root is almost as broad as the mesial root and is flattened on the distal surface. The distal root tapers more at the apical end than does the mesial root.

Occlusal Aspect

The occlusal aspect of the primary mandibular second molar is somewhat rectangular (see Figs. 3.24D and 3.29, 4). The three buccal cusps are similar in size. The two lingual cusps are also equally matched. However, the total mesiodistal width of the lingual cusps is less than the total mesiodistal width of the three buccal cusps.

Well-defined triangular ridges extend occlusally from each one of these cusp tips. The triangular ridges end in the center of the crown buccolingually in a *central developmental groove* that follows a staggered course from the *mesial triangular fossa*, just inside the *mesial marginal ridge*, to the distal triangular fossa, just mesial to the distal marginal ridge. The distal triangular fossa is not as well defined as the mesial triangular fossa. Developmental grooves branch off from the central groove both buccally and lingually, dividing the cusps. The two **buccal grooves** are confluent with the buccal developmental grooves of the buccal surface, one *mesial* and one *distal*, and the single *lingual developmental groove* is confluent with the lingual groove on the lingual surface of the crown.

Scattered over the occlusal surface are supplemental grooves on the slopes of triangular ridges and in the mesial and distal triangular fossae. The mesial marginal ridge is better developed and more pronounced than the distal marginal ridge. The outline of the crown converges distally. An outline following the tips of the cusps and the marginal ridges conforms to the outline of a rectangle more closely than does the gross outline of the crown in its entirety.

A comparison occlusally between the deciduous mandibular second molar and the permanent mandibular first molar brings out the following points of difference. In the deciduous molar, the mesiobuccal, distobuccal, and distal cusps are almost equal in size and development. The distal cusp of the permanent molar is smaller than the other two. Because of the small buccal cusps, the deciduous tooth crown is narrower buccolingually, in comparison with its mesiodistal measurement, than is the permanent tooth.

Pretest Answers

1. D
2. B
3. C
4. A
5. D

References

1. Fulton JT, Hughes JT, Mercer CV: *The life cycle of the human teeth,* Chapel Hill, NC, 1964, Department of Epidemiology, School of Public Health, University of North Carolina.
2. McBeath EC: New concept of the development and calcification of the teeth, *J Am Dent Assoc* 23:675, 1936.
3. Noyes EB, Shour I, Noyes HJ: *Dental histology and embryology,* ed 5, Philadelphia, 1938, Lea & Febiger.
4. Finn SB: *Clinical pedodontics,* ed 2, Philadelphia, 1957, Saunders.

Bibliography

Barker BC: Anatomy of root canals: IV. Deciduous teeth, *Aust Dent J* 20:101, 1975.

Baume LJ: Physiologic tooth migration and its significance for the development of occlusion. I. The biogenetic course of the deciduous dentition, *J Dent Res* 29:123, 1950.

Broadbelt AG: On the growth pattern of the human head, from the third month to the eighth year of life, *Am J Anat* 68:209, 1941.

Carlsen O: Carabelli's structure on the human maxillary deciduous first molar, *Acta Odontol Scand* 26:395, 1968.

Carlsen O, Andersen J: On the anatomy of the pulp chamber and root canals in human deciduous teeth, *Tandlaegebladet* 70:93, 1966.

de Campos Russo M, et al.: Observations on the pulpal floor of human deciduous teeth and possible implications in endodontic treatment, *Rev Fac Odontol Aracatuba* 3:61, 1974.

Fanning EA: Effect of extraction of deciduous molars on the formation and eruption of their successors, *Angle Orthod* 32:44, 1962.

Friel S: The development of ideal occlusion of the gum pads and the teeth, *Am J Orthod* 40:196, 1954.

Friel S: Occlusion: observations on its development from infancy to old age, *Int J Orthod Oral Surg* 13:322, 1927.

Moorrees CFA, Chadha M: Crown diameters of corresponding tooth groups in the deciduous and permanent dentition, *J Dent Res* 41:466, 1962.

Richardson AS, Castaldi CR: Dental development during the first two years of life, *J Can Dent Assoc* 33:418, 1967.

Van der Linden FPGM, Duterloo HS: *Development of the human dentition: an atlas,* Hagerstown, MD, 1976, Harper & Row.

Woo RK, et al.: Accessory canals in deciduous molars, *J Int Assoc Dent Child* 12:51, 1981.

4

Forensics, Comparative Anatomy, Geometries, and Form and Function

LEARNING OBJECTIVES

1. Correctly define and pronounce the new terms as emphasized in the bold type.
2. Discuss how dental anatomy and physiology may be used in forensic science
3. List two differences and two similarities when comparing human dentition with other vertebrates.
4. Draw the geometric outline form for all permanent tooth crowns from facial, lingual, mesial/distal, and incisal/occlusal views.
5. Discuss the importance of interproximal form, root form, and occlusal curvatures related to the function of the permanent dentition.

Pretest Questions

1. When viewed from the facial or lingual, the outline of all teeth may be described as which of the following shapes?
   A. Triangle
   B. Trapezoid
   C. Rhombus
   D. None of the above
2. Statement 1: The width of the occlusal table of maxillary molars is less than the width at the cervical when these teeth are viewed from the mesial or distal. Statement 2: This allows for mastication forces to be directed into a bolus of food more easily.
   A. Statement 1 and 2 are true as written.
   B. Statement 1 is true whereas statement 2 is false as written.
   C. Statement 1 is false whereas statement 2 is true as written.
   D. Statements 1 and 2 are false as written.
3. When viewed from the mesial or distal, the outline of the maxillary posterior teeth may be described as which of the following shapes?
   A. Triangle
   B. Trapezoid
   C. Rhombus
   D. None of the above
4. Which of the following is not a true statement?
   A. The gingiva within the interproximal space is called the interdental papilla.
   B. The gingival line follows the curvature of the cervical line.

   C. The cervical line is defined as the cementoenamel junction (CEJ).
   D. The gingiva normally stops at the CEJ and does not extend onto the crown.
5. When viewed from the mesial or distal, the outline of the mandibular posterior teeth may be described as which of the following shapes?
   A. Triangle
   B. Trapezoid
   C. Rhombus
   D. None of the above

For additional study resources, please visit Expert Consult.

This chapter includes brief discussions of forensic dentistry, comparative dental anatomy, and some relationships of form to function in the permanent dentition. The limited space allotted to these subjects should not suggest that they lack importance. The literature on these topics is extensive, and the reader should review the references cited for additional information.

Forensic Dentistry

Forensic dentistry (odontology) is the field within the greater disciplines of dentistry and forensic science that evaluates, manages, and presents dental evidence in legal proceedings in the interest of justice.[1] Forensic dental casework often involves identification of unidentified or missing individuals, human remains, or victims of mass fatality incidents, including natural and human-made (accidental) disasters. This is accomplished by comparison of a victim's dentition and supporting structures with dental records of known individuals. The latter records may be obtained from private dental offices, prison or military dental databases, or records retained by the Federal Bureau of Investigation through its National Crime Information Center's Missing, Unidentified, and Wanted Persons files in a web environment.[2]

Forensic odontology is one of several forensic specialties, and thus the forensic dentist's role often interfaces with those of the anthropologist, criminologist, toxicologist, pathologist, and law enforcement official involved with a case. Only a brief summary is given here, with general references added to cited references for further reading.

Jaws and Teeth

Unlike the static, genetically determined friction ridges found on the human hand and foot (commonly referred to as *fingerprints* and *footprints*) each individual's dentition is fluid and changes throughout life as the deciduous teeth are exfoliated and the permanent dentition erupts. In addition, the teeth are subject to dental and periodontal disease, the oral manifestations of systemic diseases that may affect the individual, and alterations of dental structures related to techniques of restoration and replacement that are used by the dental practitioner.

Despite this potential for an ever-changing dentition, inspection of the teeth and jaws has been used as a legally accepted method of human identification. Historically significant cases resolved by examination of dental evidence include those of Revolutionary War hero Dr. Joseph Warren (1776), the prominent Boston murder victim Dr. George Parkman (1849), and Adolph Hitler (1945). Contemporary dental identification techniques have been used in other noteworthy "cold cases," including the exhumation of Lee Harvey Oswald (1981) and the identification of the remains of the last czar of Russia and his family, who were executed by the Bolsheviks after the Russian Revolution (1991 and 2008).[3]

Paramount to the success of a forensic dental comparison between antemortem and postmortem dental records is the requirement that both sets of records provide the maximum amount of dental information for analysis. Thus dentists are encouraged to document all dental anomalies, existing restorations, and missing teeth in their written, photographic, and radiographic records.

Chronologic Age

The determination of dental maturity and tooth development is considered in Chapter 2. As indicated there, the determination of chronologic age is possible with some reasonable degree of accuracy. When it is used in conjunction with evaluation of the stage of development of osseous tissues,[4] the two methods can be used to determine an estimated age for an individual less than 20 years old. This is accomplished by entering data from both methods into an electronic encyclopedia on maxillofacial, dental, and skeletal **development**.[5]

Chronologic age determination is a central issue in population studies, and racial and gender differences in tooth development and eruption patterns are acknowledged.[6,7] Dental age assessment is also important in the forensic dental evaluation of living individuals or human remains. In the latter situation, the medicolegal need for establishing age at death can be resolved by this method. In addition, aging of the dentition has been used in forensic dental casework involving estimation of age of unidentified individuals.[8,9]

Separation of victims of multiple-fatality incidents by age facilitates the narrowing of searches for eventual identification by comparison of medical and dental records. Dental evaluation of undocumented immigrants, who may present authorities with misinformation concerning their age, is important in cases in which protection of unaccompanied minors is a concern.[2] Determination of the legal *age of majority* (adulthood) is also important in situations regarding contractual, immigration, citizenship, and criminal legal issues involving undocumented immigrants.[10]

A variety of dental age estimation procedures have been used. Those relying on tooth maturation intervals can be applied in the assessment of the teeth from the fetal stage of development through adolescence.[10,11]

Estimation of the age of an individual approaching adulthood requires additional anthropologic assessment of osseous structures, including the bones of the hands and wrist, clavicles, ribs, and cervical vertebrae. At the end of dental and skeletal development, biochemical or dental postformation changes can be used to evaluate the age of an adult.[11] Dental radiographs have also been used to determine dental chronologic age of living or deceased adult individuals.[12,13] The advantage of radiographic analysis is that it does not require destruction of dental structure.

Biochemical methods include aspartic acid racemization (AAR) and carbon-14 (^{14}C) dating. The AAR method assesses the ratios of levorotatory and dextrorotatory isomers of the long-lived, metabolically stable amino acid aspartate in both living and deceased individuals to age tissues in which this substance is found. Through a racemization process, the L form of aspartic acid is slowly transformed into its stereoisomer, which is the D form of the amino acid. As enamel and dentin age, levels of the D form of aspartic acid increase in these calcified dental structures. These values can be measured and related to known levels for age estimation.[14]

Carbon dating was first described by Libby in 1949.[15] This method is used to estimate an individual's year of birth by evaluating the rate of decay and ratio of the unstable isotope of carbon (^{14}C) relative to the levels of stable carbon (^{12}C) in the enamel and organic components of the teeth. Although AAR and ^{14}C dating analyses require expensive, lengthy laboratory procedures that eliminate dental structures, combining the results of these methods enables the investigator to determine date of birth (^{14}C), age at death (AAR), and date of death.[10]

Postformation assessment of the dentition of an adult must also consider environmental and lifestyle factors that can influence the aging process. These may include, but are not limited to, disease, diet, substance abuse, extent of physical activity, and traumatic events. Gross anatomic dental alterations were first described by Gustafson in 1950.[16] He identified six postformation dental characteristics observed in ground sections of extracted teeth: (1) attrition of the occlusal or incisal surfaces, (2) degree of deposition of secondary dentin (evaluation of size of pulp chamber and canal), (3) deposition of apical cementum, (4) attachment level of the periodontium, (5) root resorption, and (6) radicular translucency. Since then, refinements to this seminal research on the number and statistical significance of these variables have produced current methods of adult age estimation, increasing the accuracy and precision of this process.[17,18] Additional studies have taken into account the individual's gender, ethnicity, and cause of death, as well as the tooth's position and restorative status.[19,20]

Based on the extensive research in this area of dental science and the significance of the clinical determination of dental age in forensic cases, guidelines and standards have been established for dental age estimation that stress the importance of understanding the specific methodologies used to age children, adolescents, and adults and the statistical analyses used to evaluate the results of such studies.[21]

Dental DNA

Each individual's unique genetic information is contained within the nuclear deoxyribonucleic acid (DNA) and mitochondrial DNA (mtDNA) molecules of their cells. Only identical twins share the same DNA. Nuclear DNA is transmitted from either parent, whereas mtDNA is derived only through a maternal route. As a unique biologic molecule, DNA offers the forensic scientist a means of positively identifying an individual when this material can be obtained from tissues or body fluids recovered at a crime scene, or from human remains or other forensic evidence, and compared with accessible antemortem DNA.

The most widely used method for forensic analysis of DNA material is the restriction fragment length polymorphism (RFLP) technique. This laboratory procedure requires the use of large amounts (>100 ng) of DNA in the analysis. The polymerase chain reaction (PCR) technique is used when this cannot be accomplished because of degradation of the DNA molecule submitted as evidence, when only small amounts (<100 pg) of DNA are available for analysis, or when the DNA sample is fragmented.[22]

The PCR method amplifies the amount of DNA available for analysis by copying a specific locus of genetic material referred to as a short tandem repeat (STR).[23] Because only small amounts of DNA evidence are required for evaluation when using PCR technology, a positive identification may still be effected when human remains have been left unburied for long periods or have been incinerated or when DNA trace evidence is obtained from direct primary sources from the victim, including saliva, blood or fluid samples, and teeth. Additional direct secondary DNA evidence may be obtained from a toothbrush, clothing, or other personal effects.[24] Indirect samples of DNA are obtained from biologic relatives of the individual to be identified.

The calcified and pulp tissues within a tooth often present the forensic scientist with the most uncontaminated and protected DNA samples for analysis. Thus even small amounts of DNA recovered from these tissues often may be analyzed using the PCR method when other means of identification have been lost or degraded as evidence.[25–27]

In addition, PCR analysis of DNA recovered from pulp tissue can be used to determine the gender of a decedent by studying the sex-linked amelogenin gene, *AMELX* or *AMELY,* which is found on the X or the Y chromosome, respectively.[28]

Bitemarks

When the dentition of a human or animal impresses the surface of an object or tissue surface during the act of biting, a bitemark patterned injury (BMPI) is often imprinted on the bitten medium (Fig. 4.1A). As with a tool mark left as forensic evidence, the pattern left by the teeth can be evaluated and compared with the dentition that allegedly caused it (see Fig. 4.1B). Whether the BMPI

involves the skin of an assault or sexual abuse victim or suspect or is found on the surface of an inanimate object, to be probative, it must have class and individual characteristics consistent with a mark caused by teeth.

Class characteristics of a bitemark include the size and shape of the pattern. In most cases, this should be consistent with the dental arch size of the suspected biter (human or animal) and retain a circular shape consisting of two half-arches (maxilla and mandible) separated by a space (temporomandibular joint [TMJ]). One arch should be larger in its greatest dimension, representing the greater arch length of the maxilla. Individual characteristics associated with a bitemark involve the patterns routinely made by specific teeth. In the human dentition, these include the following:

Maxillary central incisor—large rectangle
Mandibular incisor and maxillary lateral incisor—small rectangle
Cuspid—point or triangle (when there is incisal wear)
Maxillary cuspid—figure-eight pattern directed buccal to lingual
Mandibular cuspid—point representing the buccal cusp
Molar—not routinely seen in the patterns left by human biters

The class and individual characteristics of the teeth creating a BMPI on human skin are manifested as contusions, abrasions, and lacerations on the surface. Interpretation of the patterned injury is often complicated by tissue avulsion, multiple BMPIs, patterns representing the dentition of more than one biter, and BPMIs that are poorly defined.

It is generally accepted that no two individuals have an identical dentition, based on variations in the arrangement, spacing, size, and shape and wear of specific teeth and dental arches. Currently, however, neither quantitative values nor databases have been established for the dentition that are similar to those described for fingerprint and DNA analysis and comparison. Thus, although bitemark evidence has been admissible in the federal and state courts of the United States based on the Frye rule and decisions related to the Federal Rules of Evidence,[29,30] this evidence is often useful only in an exculpatory manner. However, in situations involving a closed population of putative biters, each having a distinctive dentition, it may still be possible to identify the actual biter rather than simply ruling out a suspect.

Guidelines have been established and are continually reviewed and revised to provide the forensic odontologist with evidence

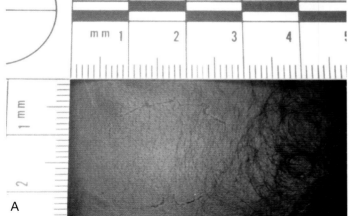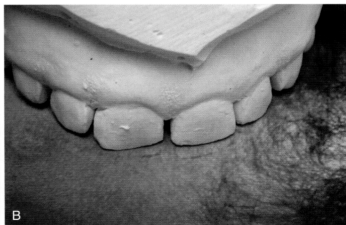

• **Fig. 4.1** Forensic bitemarks. (A) Forehead bitemarks. (B) Bitemarks related to maxillary dental cast. (Courtesy Dr. David Ord.)

gathering and analytic procedures to be followed to ensure that recovered bitemark evidence is admissible in court and supports corroborative evidence in the case.[31] Protocols have been established within these guidelines that require the forensic dental examiner to obtain admissible photographic evidence, study casts, and salivary trace evidence that may reveal the biter's DNA.[32] Criteria also have been developed defining the terms used to designate a degree of confidence that a patterned injury is a BMPI. These terms include *bitemark, suggestive of a bitemark,* and *not a bitemark.* In addition, when proffering an opinion, the forensic dental expert should, to a reasonable degree of dental certainty, use the following terms to associate a suspected biter to a bitemark:

The biter
The probable biter
Not excluded as the biter
Excluded as the biter
Inconclusive

Comparative Dental Anatomy

To understand the human dentition, it is helpful to compare the dentitions of other vertebrates. In doing so, it should become clear that the dentition in humans is different in many ways from that of other vertebrates in form and function. However, it should be equally clear that the presence of related characteristics in a wide range of vertebrates suggests a plan common to all.

Only a brief summary of the topic is presented here, starting with a simple form of tooth, the single cone or lobe, and then combinations of lobes forming more complicated teeth that are found in highly developed animals and in humans. Additional material on the subject may be found in the references and bibliography presented at the end of this chapter.

Fig. 4.2 graphically illustrates a theory of the following four phylogenetic classes of tooth forms:[33-35]
1. Single cone (haplodont)
2. Three cusps in line (triconodont)
3. Three cusps in a triangle (tritubercular molar)
4. Four cusps in a quadrangle (quadritubercular molar)

The haplodont class is represented schematically by the simplest form of tooth, the single cone (see Fig. 4.2A). This type of dentition usually includes many teeth in both jaws and is seen where jaw movements are limited to simple open and close (hinge) movements (Fig. 4.3). No occlusion of the teeth occurs in this class, because the teeth are used mainly for prehension or combat.[26,27,36,37] Their main function is the procurement of food. Jaw movements are related to and governed by tooth form in all cases.

The triconodont class exhibits three cusps in line in posterior teeth, as indicated in Fig. 4.2B. Anthropologically, the largest cusp is centered, with a smaller cusp located anteriorly and another posteriorly. Purely triconodont dentitions are not seen, although certain breeds of dogs[28,38] and other carnivores have teeth reflecting the triconodont form (Fig. 4.4). Nevertheless, dogs and other animals carnivorous by nature are considered to be in the third category (Figs. 4.5 through 4.8), the tritubercular class.[29,30,39,40] The three-cusp arrangement of the triconodont class and the more efficient three-cornered tritubercular molar arrangement are both consistent with the teeth's bypassing each other more or less when the jaw is opened or closed. However, the quadritubercular class reflects

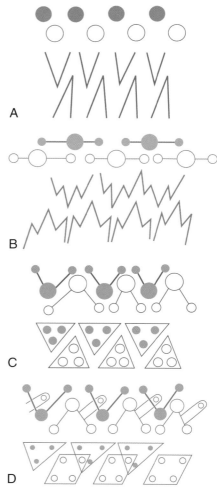

• **Fig. 4.2** Classification of cusp forms. (A) Haplodont. (B) Triconodont. (C) Tritubercular molar. (D) Quadritubercular molar. The solid dots represent upper molar cusps. The circles represent lower molar cusps. (From Thompson AH: *Comparative dental anatomy,* ed 2, revised by M Dewey, St Louis, 1915, Mosby.)

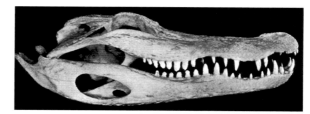

• **Fig. 4.3** The Mississippi alligator. An interesting commentary on the anatomy of the alligator: because of the alligator's physical problems, the upper jaw is the mobile one. The lower jaw, closer to the ground, is static. (From Kronfeld R: *Dental histology and comparative dental anatomy,* Philadelphia, 1937, Lea & Febiger.)

an occlusal contact relationship between the teeth of the upper and lower jaws. Articulation of the jaws and teeth is consistent with jaw movements and functions of these classes of teeth.

Animals that have dentitions similar to that of humans are anthropoid apes. This group of animals includes the chimpanzee, gibbon, gorilla, and orangutan (Figs. 4.9 and 4.10). The shapes to represent the buccal aspect of premolars or molars is turned upside down to represent the mesial or distal aspects of the same teeth. Fig. 4.16 compares maxillary parts C and D with E and F.

The fundamental considerations to be observed when reviewing the mesial or distal aspects of maxillary posterior teeth are as follows:

1. Because the occlusal surface is constricted, the tooth can be forced into food material more easily.
2. If the occlusal surface were as wide as the base of the crown, the additional chewing surface would multiply the forces of mastication.

It has been found necessary to emphasize the fundamental outlines of these aspects through the medium of schematic drawings, because the correct anatomy is overlooked so often. The tendency is to take for granted that the tooth crowns are narrowest at the cervix from all angles, which is not true. The measurement of the cervical portion of a posterior tooth is smaller than that of the occlusal portion when viewed from buccal or lingual aspects only. When it is observed from the mesial or distal aspects, the comparison is just the reverse; the occlusal surface tapers from the wide root base.

Mesial and Distal Aspects of the Mandibular Posterior Teeth

Lastly, the mandibular posterior teeth, when approached from the mesial or distal aspects, are somewhat rhomboidal in outline (see Fig. 4.16E and F). The occlusal surfaces are constricted in comparison with the bases, which is similar to the maxillary posterior teeth. The rhomboidal outline inclines the crowns lingual to the root bases, which brings the cusps into proper occlusion with the cusps of their maxillary opponents. At the same time, the axes of crowns and roots of the teeth of both jaws are kept parallel (Figs. 4.17 and 4.18). If the mandibular posterior crowns were to be set on their roots in the same relation of crown to root as that of the maxillary posterior teeth, the cusps would clash with one another. This would not allow the intercuspal relations necessary for proper function.

Summary of Schematic Outlines

Outlines of the tooth crowns, when viewed from the labial or buccal, lingual, mesial, and distal aspects, are described in a general way by triangles, trapezoids, or rhomboids (Fig. 4.16A through F).

Triangles

Six anterior teeth, maxillary and mandibular
  A. Mesial aspect
  B. Distal aspect

Trapezoids

  I. Trapezoid with longest uneven side toward occlusal or incisal surface
    A. All anterior teeth, maxillary and mandibular
      1. Labial aspect
      2. Lingual aspect
    B. All posterior teeth
      1. Buccal aspect
      2. Lingual aspect

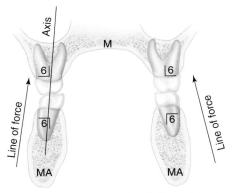

• **Fig. 4.17** Schematic representation of clinical principle of making restorations and implants consistent with directing lines of forces parallel with long axes of the teeth. *M*, Maxilla; *MA*, mandible. Teeth numbered using Zsigmondy/Palmer notation.

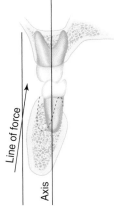

• **Fig. 4.18** Schematic representation of line of forces being incorrectly directed tangentially to the long axis of the teeth. An acceptable clinical method to determine force vectors has yet to be established.

  II. Trapezoid with shortest uneven side toward occlusal surface
    A. All maxillary posterior teeth
      1. Mesial aspect
      2. Distal aspect

Rhomboids

All mandibular posterior teeth
  A. Mesial aspect
  B. Distal aspect

Form and Function of the Permanent Dentition

The relationship between the form of the teeth and function is usually discussed in terms of type of food in the diet of humans, jaw movements, and protection of the periodontium and stimulation of the gingiva. It is also recognized that the teeth not only contribute to the digestion of food but also are important in speech and personal appearance.

The primary function of the teeth is to prepare food for swallowing and to facilitate digestion. The teeth have their respective forms to facilitate prehension, incision, and trituration of food. The dentition, joints, and muscles in humans have the form and alignment to enable the mastication of both animal and vegetable foods. This type of dentition is referred to as **omnivorous**.

The shapes of incisal and occlusal surfaces of the teeth are related not only to the function they perform but also to the movements of the mandible required to carry out chewing of a variety of foods. In contrast to the facts regarding many animals, only up-and-down jaw closure is possible because of the interlocking conical form of the teeth, TMJ morphology, and lack of muscles to carry out lateral movements. To understand more completely the form and function of teeth, the protective aspects of form and their functional relationships are considered.

Alignment, Contacts, and Occlusion

When the teeth in the mandibular arch come into contact with those in the maxillary arch in any **functional relation**, they are said to be "in occlusion." The term *occlusion* is also used to designate the anatomic alignment of the teeth and their relationship to the rest of the masticatory system. *Malocclusion* is a term usually used to describe deviations in intramaxillary and/or intermaxillary relations of the teeth and/or jaws. Occlusion is considered in more detail in Chapter 16.

As demonstrated in Chapter 1, especially relative to Table 1.1, a very low probability exists of drawing at random one tooth of each class and type from a large sample of natural teeth with the expectation of being able to place them in proper alignment and articulation, as in Figs. 1.16 through 1.18. This fact should indicate the complexity of the process of development and eruption of the teeth into a normal occlusion, which means minimally the proper alignment and arrangement of the teeth within each jaw and the interdigitation of the teeth between the jaws.[42] In addition, each tooth (including implants) in the arch should be placed in its most advantageous angle to withstand the forces brought to bear on it. The angles of the teeth are considered in Chapter 16 (see Fig. 16.20).

A general restorative principle states that occlusal forces in dental restorations should be directed along the long axis of the teeth (see Fig. 4.17). Although this concept seems appropriate, it is not **evidence based** (i.e., no appropriately designed, randomized clinical trial [RCT] results support or verify the concept). Unfortunately, currently, no acceptable method of testing the hypothesis is available (i.e., no dynamic clinical biomechanical method, including telemetry, has determined the vector forces generated between teeth during function). However, some evidence suggests that tangential loading (see Fig. 4.18) results in reduced chewing forces and that negative feedback from receptors in the periodontium mediate chewing forces. Receptor thresholds for axially directed forces appear to be higher than those for tangentially directed forces and suggest a positive feedback control on axially directed tooth forces. To position dental implants correctly, an intraoral appliance is used to guide the placement of the implant into a position and angulation consistent with angulations of opposing teeth or those suggested in Box 16.1 and Fig. 16.20.

The buccal and lingual contours of the teeth influence the way in which food is directed to and away from the gingival tissues. When a tooth is normally positioned, the gingival margin and sulcus have a physiologic relationship to the tooth in function. Food impaction, impinging trauma from tough foods, and accumulation of dental plaque may be the consequence of malposed teeth or overcontouring or undercontouring of restorations involving buccolingual surfaces. The exact relationship between the contouring of restorations and gingival health is not clear. Ideas concerning

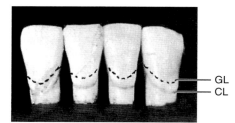

• **Fig. 4.19** The mandibular centrals and laterals contact each other at the incisal third. The form of each tooth, plus the location of the contact areas, creates narrow pointed spaces between the teeth that differ from other interproximal spaces in other segments of the arches. *CL,* Cervical line as established by the cementoenamel junction; *GL,* variable gingival line representing the gingival level.

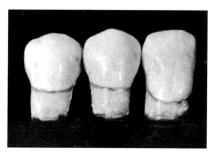

• **Fig. 4.20** Contact design and interproximal (sometimes called *interdental*) spaces illustrated by the mandibular canine and first and second premolars. Note the variation in contact areas in relation to crown length.

the relationship of faulty buccal contours (undercontouring) to the initiation of gingivitis have been challenged. Plaque control by toothbrushing may be more important than simple deviations of the contour. However, overcontoured and undercontoured restorations should be avoided. Overcontouring of facial and lingual surfaces may inhibit natural cleaning by the tongue, cheeks, and passage of food and may require special toothbrushing methods.

Interproximal Form

Proximal contacts of approximating teeth in the arch protect the soft tissues (gingiva) between the teeth and are referred to as the *interproximal spaces* (Figs. 4.19 and 4.20; see also Fig. 5.1). The gingiva, which normally fills this pyramidal-like space and extends from the alveolar bone to and around the proximal contacts of the teeth (see Fig. 5.2B), may not fill these spaces (Fig. 4.21). In the absence of correct proximal tooth contacts and marginal ridges, food impaction may occur.

The gingiva within the interproximal space is called the **gingival** or **interdental papilla** (see Fig. 5.1). Normally, the gingiva covers part of the cervical third of the tooth crowns and fills the interproximal spaces (see Figs. 4.21 and 5.1). The gingival line follows the curvature but not necessarily the level of the cervical line. The cervical line is defined as the cementoenamel junction and has been considered in Chapter 2. The gingival line and the cervical line must not be thought of as being identical; although normally following a similar curvature, these lines are seldom at the same level on the tooth. The cervical line is a stable anatomic demarcation, whereas the gingival line merely represents the gingival level on the tooth at any one period in the individual's life, and this level is variable (e.g., gingival recession). Misalignment of the

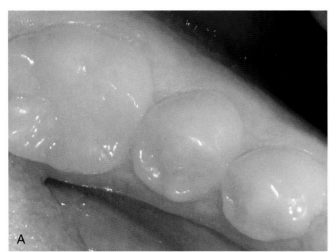

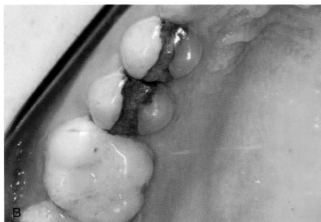

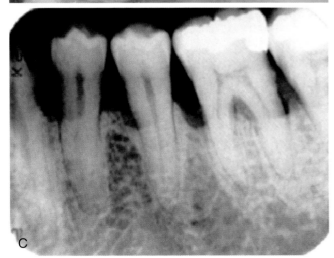

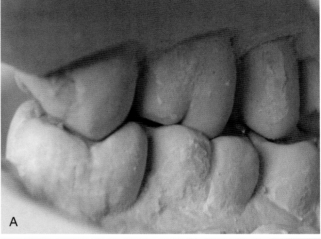

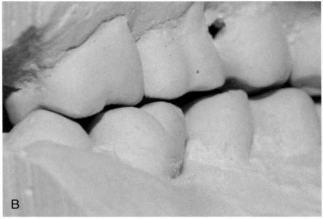

• **Fig. 5.6** Relationship of cusps to embrasures in some dentitions. (A) Casts in the intercuspal position and teeth in "normal" occlusion. (B) Other casts in intercuspal position with alignment of the teeth preventing normal contact relations between cusps and embrasure areas.

• **Fig. 5.5** Contact areas. (A) "Contacts" without evidence of dysfunction. (B) "Restored" contact areas associated with dysfunction from food impaction. (C) Loss of contacts associated with bone loss due to periodontal disease.

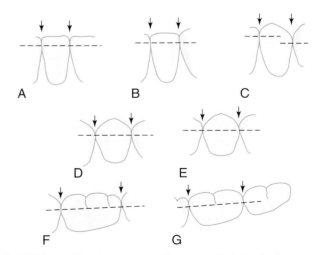

• **Fig. 5.7** Contact levels found normally on mandibular teeth. Arrows point to embrasure spaces. (A) Central and lateral incisors. (B) Central and lateral incisors and canine. (C) Lateral incisor, canine, and first premolar. (D) Canine and first and second premolars. (E), First and second premolars and first molar. (F) Second premolar and first and second molars. (G) First, second, and third molars.

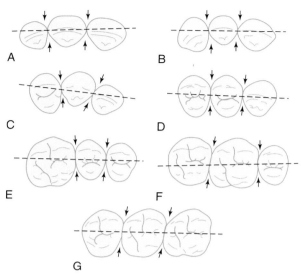

A
B
C
D
E
F
G

• **Fig. 5.8** Outline drawings of the maxillary teeth from the incisal and occlusal aspects with broken lines bisecting the contact areas. These illustrations show the relative positions of the contact areas labiolingually and buccolingually. Arrows point to embrasure spaces. (A) Central incisors and lateral incisor. (B) Central and lateral incisors and canine. (C) Lateral incisor, canine, and first premolar. (D) Canine, first premolar, and second premolar. (E) First molar, second premolar, and first molar. (F) Second premolar, first molar, and second molar. (G) First, second, and third molars.

Interproximal Spaces (Formed by Proximal Surfaces in Contact)

The interproximal spaces between the teeth are triangularly shaped spaces normally filled by **gingival** tissue (**gingival papillae**). The base of the triangle is the alveolar process, the sides of the triangle are the proximal surfaces of the contacting teeth, and the apex of the triangle is in the area of contact. The form of the interproximal space will vary with the form of the teeth in contact and will depend also on the relative position of the contact areas (Figs. 5.12 through 5.14). Normally, a separation of 1 to 1.5 mm exists between the enamel and alveolar bone. Thus the distance from the CEJ (cervical line) to the crest of the alveolar bone as seen radiographically (see Fig. 5.9) is 1 to 1.5 mm in a normal occlusion in the absence of disease.

Proper contact and alignment of adjoining teeth allows proper spacing between them for the normal bulk of gingival tissue attached to the bone and teeth. This gingival tissue is a continuation of the gingiva covering all of the alveolar process. The surface keratinization of the gingiva and the density and elasticity of the gingival tissues help to maintain these tissues against trauma during mastication and invasion by bacteria.

Because the teeth are narrower at the cervix mesiodistally than they are toward the occlusal surfaces and the outline of the root continues to taper from that point to the apices of the roots, considerable spacing is created between the roots of one tooth and the roots of adjoining teeth. This arrangement allows

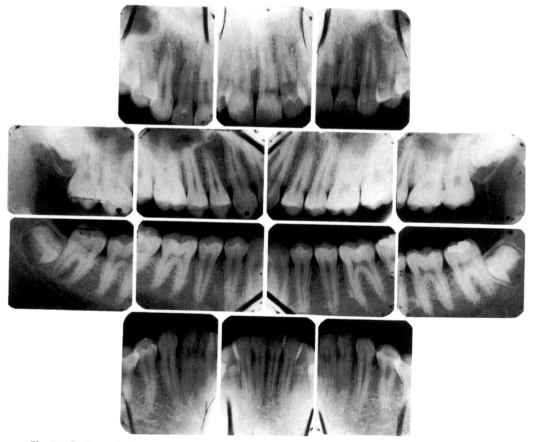

• **Fig. 5.9** Radiograph demonstrating form of alveolar crest, contact areas, and relation to form of the crown.

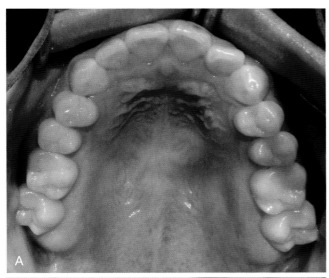

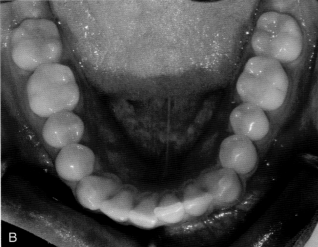

• **Fig. 5.10** Contact relations in a patient with "normal" occlusion. (A) Maxillary arch. (B) Mandibular arch.

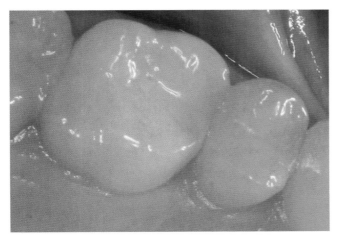

• **Fig. 5.11** Broad contact areas of the mandibular first and second molars in a young adult, 21 years old.

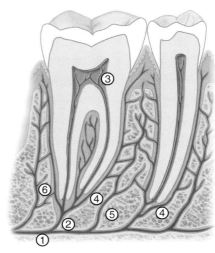

• **Fig. 5.12** Schematic drawing of distribution of the periodontal blood vessels and interdental papillae. *1,* Inferior alveolar artery; *2,* dental arteriole; *3,* pulpal branches; *4,* periodontal ligament arteriole; *5* and *6,* interalveolar arterioles. (From Ramfjord SR, Ash MM: *Periodontology and periodontics,* Philadelphia, 1979, Saunders.)

sufficient bone tissue between one tooth and another, which anchors the teeth securely in the jaws. It also simplifies the problem of space for the blood and nerve supply to the surrounding alveolar process and other investing tissues of the teeth (see Fig. 5.12).

The **type of tooth** also has a bearing on the interproximal space. Some individuals have teeth that are wide at the cervices, constricting the space at the base. Others have teeth that are more slender at the cervices than usual; this type of tooth widens the space. Teeth that are oversize or unusually small will likewise affect the interproximal spacing. Nevertheless, this spacing conforms to a plan that is fairly uniform, provided that the anatomic form is normal and the teeth are in good alignment.

Embrasures (Spillways)

When two teeth in the same arch are in contact, their curvatures adjacent to the contact areas form spillway spaces called **embrasures**. The spaces that widen out from the area of contact labially or buccally and lingually are called *labial* or *buccal* and **lingual interproximal** embrasures. These embrasures are continuous with the interproximal spaces between the teeth (see Fig. 5.10). Above the contact areas incisally and occlusally, the spaces, which are bounded by the marginal ridges as they join the cusps and incisal ridges, are called the **incisal** or **occlusal embrasures**. These embrasures, and the labial or buccal and lingual embrasures, are continuous (Fig. 5.15; see also Fig. 5.8). The curved proximal surfaces of the contacting teeth roll away from the contact area at all points, occlusally, labially or buccally, and lingually and cervically, and the embrasures and interproximal spaces are continuous, as they surround the areas of contact.

The form of embrasures serves two purposes: (1) it provides a spillway for food during mastication, a physiologic form that reduces the forces brought to bear on the teeth during the reduction of any material that offers resistance; and (2) it prevents food from being forced through the contact area. When teeth wear

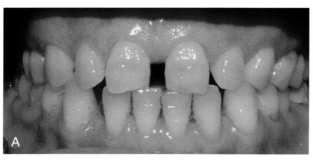

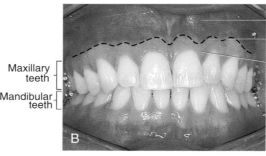

Alveolar mucosa
Mucogingival junction
Attached gingiva

Maxillary teeth
Mandibular teeth

• **Fig. 5.13** The form of the gingiva is related to the form of the teeth, contact areas, spacing between the teeth, and effects of periodontal disease and dental caries. (A) Interdental papillae do not fill the interproximal areas in several places because of spacing between the teeth. (B) Clinically normal gingivae; the form is different because of the form of the teeth, including contact areas. (From Rehrenbach MJ, Herring SW: *Illustrated Anatomy of the Head and Neck*, ed. 3, Philadelphia, 2007, W.B. Saunders.)

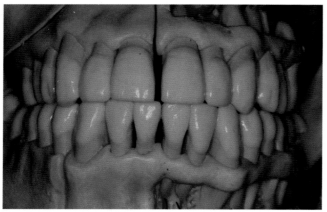

• **Fig. 5.14** The form of the teeth, position and wear of contact areas, type of teeth, and level of eruption of the teeth determine the form of the interproximal "spaces." These factors also determine the interproximal shape of the crest of alveolar bone. (Model courtesy Marcus Sommer SOMSO Modelle GmbH.)

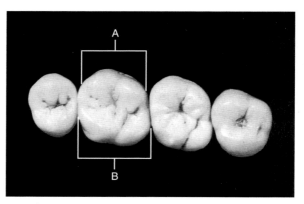

• **Fig. 5.16** Calibration of maxillary first molar. (A) Calibration at prominent buccal line angles that functions by deflecting food material during mastication. (B) Calibration of lingual contour from contact area mesially to contact area distally. There are no prominent line angles, but the development of the mesiolingual cusp has widened the rounded lingual form. Thus the two lingual embrasures are kept similar in size, even though the tooth makes contact with two teeth that are dissimilar lingually. This way, the lingual gingival tissue interproximally is properly protected by the equalization of lingual embrasures.

down to the contact area so that no embrasure remains, especially in the incisors, food is pushed into the contact area even when teeth are not mobile.

The design of contact areas, interproximal spaces, and embrasures varies with the form and alignment of the various teeth; each section of the two arches shows similarity of form. In other words, the contact form, the interproximal spacing, and the embrasure form seem rather constant in sectional areas of the dental arches. These sections are named as follows: the maxillary anterior section, the mandibular anterior section, the maxillary posterior section, and the mandibular posterior section. All embrasure spaces are reflections of the form of the teeth involved. Maxillary central and lateral incisors exhibit one embrasure form, the mandibular incisors another, and so on.

Maxillary posteriors and mandibular posteriors apparently require an embrasure design geared for their sections. In some cases the constancy has to be attained by a tooth form adaptation (Fig. 5.16). For instance, the canines are shaped so that they act as a catalyst in these matters between anterior and posterior teeth. A line bisecting the labial portion of either canine seems to create

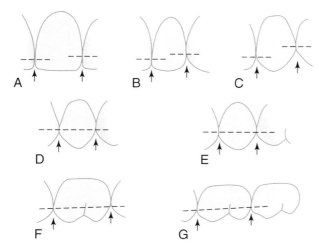

• **Fig. 5.15** Outline drawings of the maxillary teeth in contact, with dotted lines bisecting the contact areas at the various levels as found normally. Arrows point to embrasure spaces. (A) Central and lateral incisors. (B) Central and lateral incisors and canine. (C) Lateral incisor, canine, and first premolar. (D) Canine and first and second premolars. (E) First and second premolars and first molar. (F) Second premolar, first molar, and second molar. (G) First, second, and third molars. (To view Animations 5 and 6, please go to Expert Consult.)

an anterior half mesially that resembles half of an anterior tooth and a posterior half that resembles a posterior tooth. The mesial contact is at one level for contact with the lateral incisor, but the distal contact form must be at a level consistent with the contact form of the first premolar, whether maxillary or mandibular (see Fig. 5.15C).

Contact Areas and Incisal and Occlusal Embrasures From the Labial and Buccal Aspect

It is advisable to refer continually to the illustrations of contacts and embrasures during the reading of the descriptions that follow. Locate the illustration of interest (see Fig. 5.15A) while reading the details concerning contact area levels in the following paragraphs.

Maxillary Teeth

Central Incisors
The contact areas mesially on both central incisors are located at the incisal third of the crowns. Because the mesioincisal third of these teeth approaches a right angle, the incisal embrasure is very slight.

Central and Lateral Incisors
The distal outline of the central incisor crown is rounded. The lateral incisor has a shorter crown and has a more rounded mesioincisal angle than the central incisor. The form of these two teeth coming into contact with each other therefore opens up an embrasure space distal to the central incisors larger than the small one mesial to the central incisors. A line bisecting the contact areas distal to the central incisor and mesial to the lateral incisor approaches the junction of the middle and incisal thirds of each crown.

Lateral Incisor and Canine
The distal contact area on the lateral incisor is approximately at the middle third. The mesial contact area on the canine is at the junction of the incisal and middle thirds. The form of these teeth creates an embrasure that is more open than the two previously described.

Canine and First Premolar
The canine has a long distal slope to its cusp, which puts the distal crest of curvature at the center of the middle third of the crown. The contact area is therefore at that point. This is an important observation to be made clinically. As mentioned, it is at this point in the dental arch that the canine, situated between the anterior and posterior segments, becomes a part of both (see Fig. 5.15B and C).

The first premolar has a long cusp form also, which puts its mesial contact area rather high up on the crown. Usually it is just cervical to the junction of the occlusal and middle thirds. The embrasure between these teeth has a wide angle.

First and Second Premolars
The contact areas of the first and second premolars are similar to those just mentioned, although usually a little cervical to the junction of the occlusal and middle thirds of the crowns. The form of these teeth creates a wide occlusal embrasure.

Note that the design of the interproximal spaces changes also with the form and dimensions of the teeth in contact.

Second Premolar and First Molar
The position of the second premolar and first molar contact areas cervico-occlusally is approximately the same as that found between the premolars.

First and Second and Second and Third Molars
The two contact and embrasure forms for the first and second and second and third molars may be described together because they are similar. The distal outline of the first molar is round, a fact that puts the contact area approximately at the center of the middle third of the crown. Here again, it must be emphasized that contact levels on maxillary molars (and even on premolars to some extent) tend to be centered in the middle third of the anatomical crown.

The mesial contact area of the second molar also approaches the middle third of the crown. The occlusal embrasure is generous as a consequence, even though the cusps are not long.

The contact and embrasure design of the second and third molars is similar to that of the first and second molars. The molars become progressively shorter from the first through the third. Again, the dimensions of the tooth crowns affect the contact and embrasure design.

Mandibular Teeth

Central Incisors
The mesial contact areas on the mandibular central incisors are located at the incisal third of the crowns. At the time of the eruption of these teeth, the mesial and distal incisal angles are slightly rounded, and the mamelons are noticeable on the incisal ridges. However, soon incisal wear reduces the incisal ridge to a straight surface, and the mesial and distal angles approach right angles in sharpness. This is due partly to wear at the contact areas (see Figs. 5.7 and 5.14). In many instances, the contact areas extend to the mesioincisal angle. Therefore a small incisal embrasure occurs mesially between the mandibular central incisors unless wear through use obliterates it.

Central and Lateral Incisors
The distal contact areas and the incisal embrasures on the central incisors and the mesial contact areas and incisal embrasures on the lateral incisors are similar to those just described. Because the mandibular central and lateral incisors are small mesiodistally and supplement each other in function, the design of their crowns brings about similar contact and embrasure forms.

Note the slender Gothic arch–like spaces that circumscribe the interproximal spaces between the mandibular anterior teeth.

Lateral Incisor and Canine
The positions of the contact areas distally on the lateral incisor and mesially on the canine are approximately the same, cervicoincisally, as the other two just described. The teeth are in contact at the incisal third close to the incisal ridges. However, the mesioincisal angle of the canine is more rounded than the others, which opens up a small incisal embrasure at this point.

The interproximal spacing between lateral and canine is very similar in outline to the two interproximal spaces just described.

Canine and First Premolar
The distal slope of the cusp of the mandibular canine is pronounced and long, which places the distal contact area on this tooth somewhat cervical to the junction of its incisal and middle thirds.

The first premolar has a long buccal cusp, and although its crown is shorter than that of the canine, the mesial contact area has approximately the same relation cervico-occlusally as that found distally on the canine and is just cervical to the junction of the occlusal and middle thirds. Thus the whole arrangement places these contact areas level with each other.

The occlusal embrasure is quite wide and pronounced because of the cusp forms of the two teeth. The interproximal space has been reduced by the lowering of the contact areas cervically, comparing favorably to the design for posterior mandibular teeth.

First and Second Premolars

From the buccal aspect, the crowns of the first and second premolars are similar. The buccal cusp of the second premolar is not quite as long as that of the first premolar. The contact of these teeth is nearly level with that of the canine and first premolar. The slope of the cusps creates a large occlusal embrasure. The interproximal space is a little smaller than that between the canine and first premolar.

Second Premolar and First Molar

The contact and embrasure design for the second premolar and first molar is similar to that just described for the premolars. The mesiobuccal cusp of the first molar is shorter and more rounded than the cusp of the second premolar, which varies the embrasure somewhat, and because the crown of the molar is a little shorter, it reduces the interproximal space to that extent.

First and Second and Second and Third Molars

The two contact and embrasure designs of the first and second and second and third molars may be described together because they are similar.

The proximal surfaces (i.e., the distal surface of the first molar, mesial surface of the second molar, distal surface of the second molar, and mesial surface of the third molar) are quite round. The occlusal embrasures are therefore generous above the points of contact, even though the cusps are short and rounded.

Because the molars become progressively shorter from the first to the third, the centers of the contact areas also drop cervically. A line bisecting the contact areas of the second and third molars is located approximately at the center of the middle thirds of the crowns.

The interproximal spaces have been reduced considerably because of their shortened form.

Contact Areas and Labial, Buccal, and Lingual Embrasures From the Incisal and Occlusal Aspects

To study the relative positions of contact areas and the related labial, buccal, and lingual embrasures and also to get proper perspective, the eye must be directed at the incisal surfaces of anterior teeth and directly above the surface of each tooth being examined in series (Fig. 5.17; see also Figs. 5.8, 5.10, and 5.11). Posterior teeth are examined in the same manner. Look down on each tooth or group of teeth by facing the occlusal surfaces on a line with the long axis.

The problem at this point is to discover the relative positions of contacts in a labiolingual or buccolingual direction and to observe

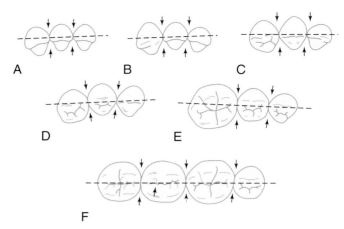

• **Fig. 5.17** Contact relation of mandibular teeth labiolingually and buccolingually when surveyed from the incisal and occlusal aspects. Arrows point to embrasure spaces. (A) Central incisors and lateral incisor. (B) Central and lateral incisors and canine. (C) Lateral incisor, canine, and first premolar. (D) Canine, first premolar, and second premolar. (E) First premolar, second premolar, and first molar. (F) Second premolar and first, second, and third molars.

the embrasure form facially and lingually created by the tooth forms and their contact relations.

A generalization may be established in locating contact areas faciolingually. Anterior teeth will have their contacts centered labiolingually, whereas posterior teeth will have contact areas slightly buccal to the center buccolingually. This buccal inclination must be carefully studied and must not be overemphasized.

Except for the maxillary first molar, all crowns converge more lingually than facially from contact areas. The maxillary first molar is the only tooth wider lingually than buccally (see Fig. 5.16). Its formation makes a necessary adjustment of the mesiolingual embrasure when the tooth form of maxillary posteriors changes from the maxillary premolar form to the purely rhomboidal form of maxillary second and third molars. This situation is discussed more fully later.

The narrower measurement lingually rather than facially causes wider embrasures lingually compared with facial embrasures. Compare the two types of embrasures displayed by maxillary central and lateral incisors.

Maxillary Teeth

See Figs. 5.8 and 5.10A.

Central Incisors

The contact areas of the central incisors are centered labiolingually. The labial embrasure is a V-shaped space created by the labial form of these crowns. The lingual embrasure widens out more than the labial embrasure because of the lingual convergence of the crowns (see Fig. 5.10A). Note the centering of the labioincisal edge with respect to the crown outline of these teeth and the narrowness of the lingual surfaces in comparison with the broad labial faces.

Central and Lateral Incisors

The contact areas of the central and lateral teeth are centered labiolingually also.

Lateral Incisor and Canine

The contact area of the lateral incisor and canine is centered labiolingually on both canine and lateral incisors. The lingual embrasure is similar to that of the central and lateral incisors, but the labial embrasure is changed somewhat by a definite convexity at the mesiolabial line angle of the canine.

Canine and First Premolar

The contact area of the canine and first premolar is centered on the distal surface of the canine but is a little buccal to the center on the mesial surface of the first premolar. The embrasure design lingually is marked by a concavity in the region of the distolingual line angle of the canine and by a developmental groove crossing the mesial marginal ridge of the first premolar.

First and Second Premolars

The contact areas of the first and second premolars are nearly centered buccolingually. The embrasures buccally and lingually are regular in outline, although slightly different in design.

The prominence of the mesiobuccal and distobuccal line angles of the premolars is in direct contrast to the even taper of these teeth lingually, as viewed from the occlusal aspect. This form demonstrates a slight variation between buccal and lingual embrasures.

Second Premolar and First Molar

As usual, a line bisecting the contact areas of the second premolar and first molar is nearly centered on the distal surface of the second premolar. The area on the mesial surface of the first molar is located farther buccally than other contact areas on the maxillary posterior teeth. The contact areas are wider on molars because of the greater width buccolingually of the molar teeth.

The buccal embrasure between these teeth and the location of the mesial contact area of the first molar are influenced by the prominence of the mesiobuccal line angle of the maxillary first molar and the matching prominence of the distobuccal line angle of the maxillary second premolar. The lingual embrasure is kept standard for the molar area by the enlargement of the mesiolingual cusp of the first molar. Occasionally, this cusp carries a small conformation lingually as part of the change in form (fifth cusp, or cusp of Carabelli). Usually, the mesiolingual cusp of the maxillary first molar is rounded out, with no more than a developmental groove showing that an extra cusp formation may have been intended.

However, the mesiolingual lobe of this tooth is always large, causing the tooth to be wider lingually from its mesiolingual line angle to its distolingual line angle than it is from the mesiobuccal line angle to the distobuccal line angle. If it were not for this fact, the rhomboid form of the first molar in contact with the tapered form of the second premolar would open up a lingual embrasure of extremely large proportions. The large mesiolingual lobe makes up for the change in occlusal outline from premolar form to molar form, keeping the conformity of the lingual embrasures (see Fig. 5.16).

First and Second and Second and Third Molars

The contact and embrasure forms of the first and second and second and third molars may be described together because they are similar. Although the mesiobuccal line angles of the second and third molars are not as sharp as that of the first molar, they are prominent nevertheless.

The distobuccal line angles of all the maxillary molars are indistinct and rounded, so that the buccal embrasure forms are shaped and characterized mainly by the prominent mesiobuccal line angle. The mesiolingual line angles of the second and third molars are rounded and in conjunction with the rounded distolingual line angles; the lingual embrasures between first, second, and third molars present a regular and open form (see Fig. 5.8F and G).

The contact areas are broad and centered buccolingually. The embrasures are uniform. Note the generous proportions of the buccal embrasures.

Mandibular Teeth

See Figs. 5.10, 5.11, and 5.17.

Central Incisors and Central and Lateral Incisors

The contact areas and embrasures of the central incisors and the central and lateral incisors may be described together because they are similar.

Although these teeth are narrow mesiodistally, their labiolingual measurements are not much less than those of the maxillary central and lateral incisors. The mandibular central incisors come within a millimeter or so of having the same labiolingual diameter as that of the maxillary central incisors; the *mandibular* lateral incisors have a labiolingual diameter as great if not greater than that of the *maxillary* lateral incisors.

The contact areas are centered labiolingually, and the embrasures are uniform. Although the mesiodistal dimensions are less, the outline form of the incisal aspects of the mandibular central and lateral incisors is similar to that of the maxillary central and lateral incisors in that the lingual outlines have a rounded taper in comparison with broader, flattened labial faces.

Lateral Incisor and Canine

The contact areas of the lateral incisor and canine are centered, and the lingual embrasure is similar to those just described. The labial embrasure is influenced by the prominence of the mesiolabial line angle of the canine. Note that the maxillary canine presents the same characteristic.

Canine and First Premolar

The canine and first premolar contact areas are approximately centered, and the buccal embrasure is smooth and uniform in outline. The lingual embrasure is opened up somewhat by a slight concavity on the canine distolingually and by a characteristic developmental groove across the marginal ridge of the first premolar mesiolingually.

First and Second Premolars

The contact areas of the first and second premolars are nearly centered buccolingually but are broader than those found mesial to them, because the distal curvature of the first premolar describes a larger arc than the mesial curvature and the mesial contacting surface of the second premolar is relatively broad and describes a shallower curved surface than that of the distal surface of the first premolar.

Because of the lingual convergence of the first premolar and the narrow lingual cusp form, the lingual embrasure is as wide as the one mesial to it.

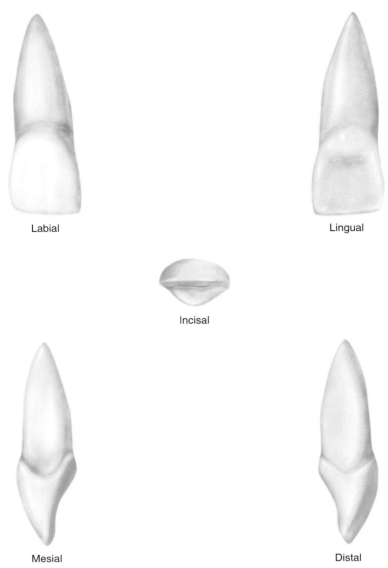

Labial

Lingual

Incisal

Mesial

Distal

• **Fig. 6.8** Maxillary right central incisor.

The distal outline of the crown is more convex than the mesial outline, with the crest of curvature higher toward the cervical line. The distoincisal angle is not as sharp as the mesioincisal angle, the extent of curvature depending on the typal form of the tooth.

The incisal outline is usually regular and straight in a mesiodistal direction after the tooth has been in function long enough to obliterate the mamelons. The incisal outline tends to curve downward toward the center of the crown outline, so that the crown length is greater at the center than at the two mesial angles.

The cervical outline of the crown follows a semicircular direction with the curvature rootwise, from the point at which the root outline joins the crown mesially to the point at which the root outline joins the crown distally.

The root of the central incisor from the labial aspect is cone shaped, in most instances with a relatively blunt apex, and the outline mesially and distally is regular. The root is usually 2 or 3 mm longer than the crown, although it varies considerably (see illustrations of typical central incisors and those of variations from the labial aspects in Figs. 6.9 and 6.12).

A line drawn through the center of the root and crown of the maxillary central incisor tends to parallel the mesial outline of the crown and root.

Lingual Aspect

The lingual outline of the maxillary central incisor is the reverse of that found on the labial aspect (see Fig. 6.3). However, the lingual aspect of the crown is different when we compare the surface of the lingual aspect with that of the labial aspect. From the labial aspect, the surface of the crown is smooth generally. The lingual aspect has convexities and a concavity. The outline of the cervical line is similar, but immediately below the cervical line a smooth convexity is to be found; this is called the **cingulum** (see Fig. 6.1).

Mesially and distally confluent with the cingulum are the **marginal ridges.** Between the marginal ridges, below the cingulum, a shallow concavity is present called the **lingual fossa.** Outlining the lingual fossa, the linguoincisal edge is raised somewhat, being on a level with the marginal ridges mesially and distally, completing the lingual portion of the incisal ridge of the central incisor.

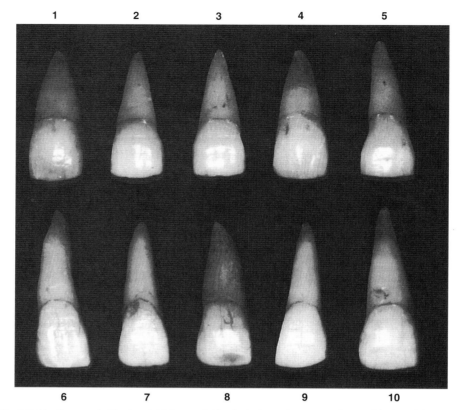

• **Fig. 6.9** Maxillary central incisor, labial aspect. Ten typical specimens are shown. (To view Animations 3 and 4 for tooth #8, please go to Expert Consult.)

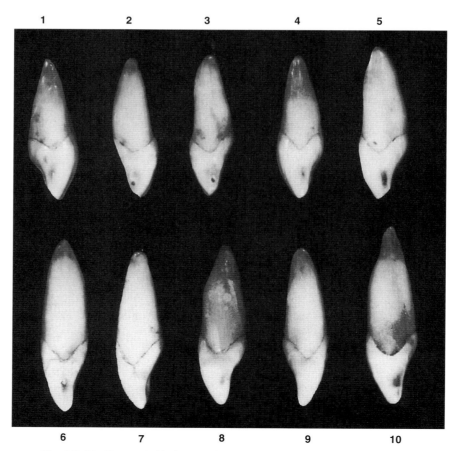

• **Fig. 6.10** Maxillary central incisor, mesial aspect. Ten typical specimens are shown.

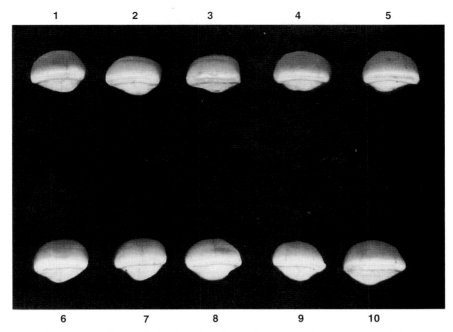

• **Fig. 6.11** Maxillary central incisor, incisal aspect. Ten typical specimens are shown.

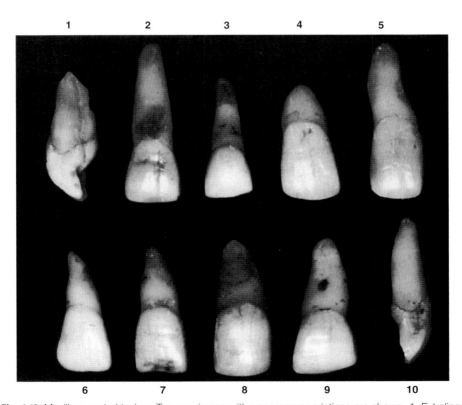

• **Fig. 6.12** Maxillary central incisor. Ten specimens with uncommon variations are shown. *1,* Extralingual inclination of incisal portion of crown. Note developmental (palatoradicular) groove traversing root and part of crown. *2,* Root extremely long. *3,* Specimen small in all dimensions. *4,* Crown extremely long, root very short. *5,* Specimen malformed; crown unusually long; cervix very wide. *6,* Root short and tapering. *7,* Same as specimen 6. *8,* Crown nearly as wide at the cervix as at contact areas, crown long, root short. *9,* Root with unusual curvature. *10,* Crown and root narrow labiolingually; root comparable with that of specimen 2.

TABLE 6.1	**Maxillary Central Incisor**

First evidence of calcification	3–4 months
Enamel completed	4–5 years
Eruption	7–8 years
Root completed	10 years

MEASUREMENT TABLE							
	Cervicoincisal Length of Crown	Length of Root	Mesiodistal Diameter of Crown	Mesiodistal Diameter of Crown at Cervix	Labiolingual or Buccolingual Diameter of Crown	Labiolingual or Buccolingual Diameter of Crown at Cervix	Curvature of Cervical Line—Mesial	Curvature of Cervical Line—Distal
Dimensions[a] suggested for carving technique	10.5	13.0	8.5	7.0	7.0	6.0	3.5	2.5

[a]In millimeters.

From the foregoing description, we note that the lingual fossa is bordered mesially by the mesial marginal ridge, incisally by the lingual portion of the incisal ridge, distally by the distal marginal ridge, and cervically by the cingulum. Usually there are developmental grooves extending from the cingulum into the lingual fossa.

The crown and root taper lingually, so that the crown calibration at the two labial line angles is greater than the calibration at the two lingual line angles, and the lingual portion of the root is narrower than the labial portion. A cross section of the root at the cervix shows the root to be generally triangular with rounded angles. One side of the triangle is labial, with the mesial and distal sides pointing lingually. The mesial side of this triangle is slightly longer than the distal side (see Fig. 13.8C, *3, 4, 5,* and *6*).

Mesial Aspect

The mesial aspect of this tooth has the fundamental form of an incisor. The crown is wedge shaped, or triangular, with the base of the triangle at the cervix and the apex at the incisal ridge (see Fig. 4.16A and Figs. 6.4 and 6.10).

Usually, a line drawn through the crown and the root from the mesial aspect through the center of the tooth will bisect the apex of the root and also the incisal ridge of the crown. The incisal ridge of the crown is therefore on a line with the center of the root. This alignment is characteristic of maxillary central and lateral incisors. A straight line drawn through the center of the crown and root from the mesial or distal aspects will rarely if ever pass lingual to the incisal edge. Maxillary incisors are occasionally seen with the incisal ridges lingual to the bisecting line (see Fig. 6.12, *1*).

Labially and lingually, immediately coronal to the cervical line are the crests of curvature of these surfaces. These crests of contour give the crown its greatest labiolingual measurement.

Normally, the curvature labially and lingually is approximately 0.5 mm in extent (see Fig. 6.4) before continuing the outlines to the incisal ridge.

The labial outline of the crown from the crest of curvature to the incisal ridge is very slightly convex. The lingual outline is convex at the point where it joins the crest of curvature at the cingulum; it then becomes concave at the mesial marginal ridge and slightly convex again at the linguoincisal ridge and the incisal edge.

The cervical line outlining the cementoenamel junction (CEJ) mesially on the maxillary central incisor curves incisally to a noticeable degree. This cervical curvature is greater on the mesial surface of this tooth than on any surface of any other tooth in the mouth. The curvature varies in extent, depending on the length of the crown and the measurement of the crown labiolingually. On an average central incisor of 10.5 to 11 mm in crown length, the curvature is 3 to 4 mm (see Fig. 5.26).

The root of this tooth from the mesial aspect is cone shaped, and the apex of the root is usually bluntly rounded.

Distal Aspect

Little difference is evident between the distal and mesial outlines of this tooth (see Fig. 6.5). When looking at the central incisor from the distal aspect, it may be noted that the crown gives the impression of being somewhat thicker toward the incisal third. Because of the slope of the labial surface distolingually, more of that surface is seen from the distal aspect; this creates the illusion of greater thickness. Actually, most teeth are turned a little on their root bases to adapt to the dental arch curvature. The maxillary central incisor is no exception.

The curvature of the cervical line outlining the CEJ is less in extent on the distal than on the mesial surfaces. Most teeth show this characteristic.

Incisal Aspect

The specimen of this tooth is posed in the illustrations so that the incisal edge is centered over the root (see Figs. 6.6 and 6.11). A view of the crown from this aspect superimposes it over the root entirely so that the latter is not visible.

From this aspect, the labial face of the crown is relatively broad and flat in comparison with the lingual surface, especially toward the incisal third. Nevertheless, the cervical portion of the crown labially is convex, although the arc described is broad.

The incisal ridge may be seen clearly, and a differentiation between the incisal edge and the remainder of the incisal ridge, with its slope toward the lingual, is easily distinguished.

The outline of the lingual portion tapers lingually toward the cingulum. The cingulum of the crown makes up the cervical portion of the lingual surface.

The mesiolabial and distolabial line angles are prominent from the incisal aspect. The relative positions of these line angles should be compared with the mesiolingual and distolingual line angles, which are represented by the borders of the mesial and distal marginal ridges. The mesiodistal calibration of the crown at the labial line angles is greater than the same calibration at the lingual line angles.

The crown of this tooth shows more bulk from the incisal aspect than one would expect from viewing it from the mesial or distal aspect. Relatively broad surfaces are at the site of contact areas mesially and distally. Comparison should also be made between the dimensions of the crown labiolingually and mesiodistally. The labiolingual calibration of the crown is more than two-thirds as great as the mesiodistal calibration. A cursory examination would not reveal this detail.

Bilaterally, the outline of the incisal aspect is rather uniform. However, the lingual portion shows some variation in that a line drawn from the mesioincisal angle to the center of the cingulum lingually will be longer than one drawn from the same point on the cingulum to the distoincisal angle. The crown conforms to a triangular outline reflected by the outline of the root cross section at the cervix mentioned earlier.

Maxillary Lateral Incisor

Figs. 6.13 through 6.21 illustrate the maxillary lateral incisor in various aspects. Because the maxillary lateral incisor supplements the central incisor in function, the crowns bear a close resemblance. The lateral incisor is smaller in all dimensions except root length (Table 6.2). Because it resembles the maxillary central incisor in form, direct comparisons are made with the central incisor in its description.

This tooth differs from the central incisor in its development, which may vary considerably. Maxillary lateral incisors vary in form more than any other tooth in the mouth except the third molar. If the variation is too great, it is considered a developmental anomaly.

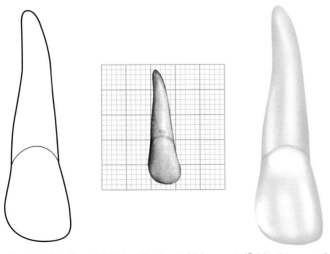

• **Fig. 6.13** Maxillary right lateral incisor, labial aspect. (Grid = 1 sq. mm.)

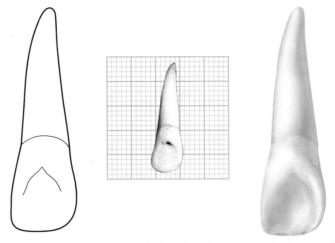

• **Fig. 6.14** Maxillary right lateral incisor, lingual aspect. (Grid = 1 sq. mm.)

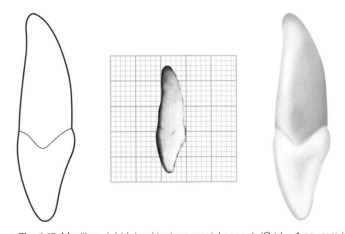

• **Fig. 6.15** Maxillary right lateral incisor, mesial aspect. (Grid = 1 sq. mm.)

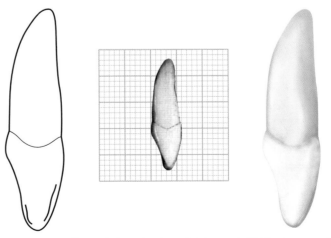

• **Fig. 6.16** Maxillary right lateral incisor, distal aspect. (Grid = 1 sq. mm.)

A common situation is to find maxillary lateral incisors with a nondescript, pointed form; such teeth are called **peg-shaped** laterals (see Fig. 6.21, *7* and *8*). In some individuals the lateral incisors are missing entirely;[7] in these cases the maxillary central incisor may

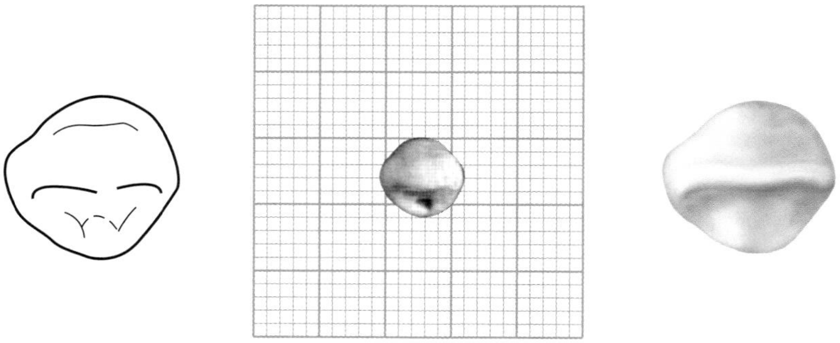

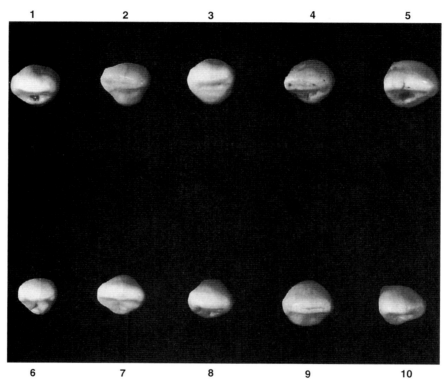

• **Fig. 6.17** Maxillary right lateral incisor, incisal aspect. (Grid = 1 sq. mm.)

• **Fig. 6.18** Maxillary lateral incisor, incisal aspect. Ten typical specimens are shown.

be in contact distally with the canine. The presence of a palatogingival groove in maxillary incisors may be a predisposing factor in localized periodontal disease (see Fig. 6.21, 3).[8] This groove is also referred to as the **palatoradicular groove.**[9]

One type of malformed maxillary lateral incisor has a large, pointed tubercle as part of the cingulum; some have deep developmental grooves that extend down on the root lingually with a deep fold in the cingulum; and some show twisted roots, distorted crowns, and so on (see Fig. 6.21).

Detailed Description of the Maxillary Lateral Incisor From All Aspects

Labial Aspect

Although the labial aspect of the maxillary lateral incisor may appear to favor that of the central incisor, usually it has more

curvature, with a rounded incisal ridge and rounded incisal angles mesially and distally (see Figs. 6.13 and 6.19). Although the crown is smaller in all dimensions, its proportions usually correspond to those of the central incisor.

The mesial outline of the crown from the labial aspect resembles that of the central incisor, with a more rounded mesioincisal angle. The crest of contour mesially is usually at the point of junction of the middle and incisal thirds; occasionally, in the so-called square forms, the mesioincisal angle is almost as sharp as that found on most maxillary central incisors (see Fig. 6.19, 4 and 5). However, a more rounded mesioincisal angle is seen more often. The distal outline of the crown from the labial aspect differs somewhat from that of the central incisor.

The distal outline is always more rounded, and the crest of contour is more cervical, usually in the center of the middle

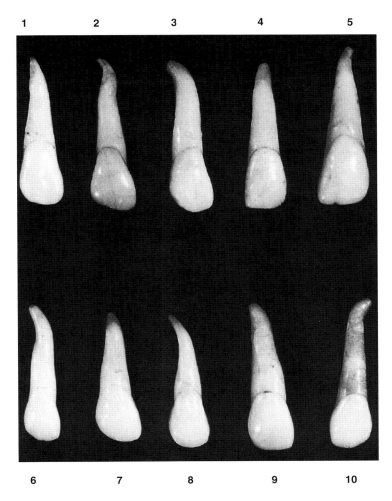

• **Fig. 6.19** Maxillary lateral incisor, labial aspect. Ten typical specimens are shown. (To view Animations 3 and 4 for tooth #7, please go to Expert Consult.)

third. Some forms describe a semicircular outline distally from the cervix to the center of the incisal ridge (see Fig. 6.19, *3* and *7*).

The labial surface of the crown is more convex than that of the central incisor except in some square and flat-faced forms.

This tooth is relatively narrow mesiodistally, usually approximately 2 mm narrower than the central incisor. The crown on the average measures from 2 to 3 mm shorter cervicoincisally than that of the central incisor, although the root is usually as long, if not somewhat longer, than that of the central incisor.

In general, its root length is greater in proportion to its crown length than that of the central incisor. The root is often approximately 1.5 times the length of the crown.

The root tapers evenly from the cervical line to a point approximately two-thirds of its length apically. In most cases, it curves sharply from this location in a distal direction and ends in a pointed apex. Although the curvature distally is typical, some roots are straight (see Fig. 6.19, *4, 7,* and *9*), and some may be found curving mesially. As mentioned previously, this tooth may show considerable variance in its crown form; the root form may be more characteristic.

Lingual Aspect

From the lingual aspect, mesial and distal marginal ridges are marked, and the cingulum is usually prominent, with a tendency toward deep developmental grooves within the lingual fossa, where it joins the cingulum (see Fig. 6.14). The linguoincisal ridge is well developed, and the lingual fossa is more concave and circumscribed than that found on the central incisor. The tooth tapers toward the lingual, resembling a central incisor in this respect. It is not uncommon to find a deep developmental groove at the side of the cingulum, usually on the distal side, which may extend up on the root for part or all of its length. Faults in the enamel of the crown are often found in the deep portions of these developmental grooves (see Fig. 6.21, *3* and *4*).

Mesial Aspect

The mesial aspect of the maxillary lateral incisor is similar to that of a small central incisor except that the root appears longer (see Figs. 6.15 and 6.20). The crown is shorter, the root is relatively longer, and the labiolingual measurement of the crown and root is a millimeter or so less than that of the maxillary central incisor of the same mouth.

TABLE 7.2	Mandibular Lateral Incisor

First evidence of calcification	3–4 months
Enamel completed	4–5 years
Eruption	7–8 years
Root completed	10 years

MEASUREMENT TABLE							
	Cervicoincisal Length of Crown	Length of Root	Mesiodistal Diameter of Crown	Mesiodistal Diameter of Crown at Cervix	Labio- or Buccolingual Diameter of Crown	Labio- or Buccolingual Diameter of Crown at Cervix	Curvature of Cervical Line, Mesial	Curvature of Cervical Line, Distal
Dimensions[a] suggested for carving technique	9.5	14.0	5.5	4.0	6.5	5.8	3.0	2.0

[a]In millimeters.

and root labiolingually, as was found when observing the central incisor; the edge follows the curvature of the mandibular dental arch, which gives the crown of the mandibular lateral incisor the appearance of being twisted slightly on its root base (see Figs. 7.17 and 7.18). It is interesting to note that the labiolingual root axes of mandibular central and lateral incisors remain almost parallel in the alveolar process, even though the incisal ridges are not directly in line. (To view Animations 3 and 4, please go to Expert Consult.)

Pretest Answers

1. A
2. C
3. A
4. A
5. C

References

1. Carlsen O: *Dental morphology*, Copenhagen, 1987, Munksgaard.
2. Pindborg JJ: *Pathology of the dental tissues*, Philadelphia, 1970, Saunders.
3. Woelfel JB, Scheid RC: *Dental anatomy: its relevance to dentistry*, ed 5, Baltimore, 1997, Williams & Wilkins.
4. Hanihara K: Racial characteristics in the dentition, *J Dent Res* 46:293, 1967.

8

The Permanent Canines: Maxillary and Mandibular

LEARNING OBJECTIVES

1. Correctly define and pronounce the new terms as emphasized in the bold type.
2. Correctly label the anatomic landmarks of permanent maxillary and mandibular canines.
3. Discuss the grid diagrams of the permanent maxillary and mandibular canines and be able to correctly draw the graph outlines of each tooth from all views. *Note: Being able to model correct tooth contours is fundamental to learning. Drawing, waxing, and/ or carving the teeth are good ways to practice this.*
4. Discuss common anatomic variations seen in each tooth type.
5. List similarities and differences between permanent maxillary and mandibular canines.

Pretest Questions

1. Calcification of the permanent mandibular canine begins at about what age?
   A. 2 to 3 months
   B. 4 to 5 months
   C. 2 to 3 years
   D. 4 to 5 years
2. The mesial contact area of the permanent maxillary canine is centered where on the crown?
   A. Incisal third
   B. Middle third
   C. Junction of the incisal and middle thirds
   D. Junction of the middle and cervical thirds
3. Which of the following teeth is most likely to have a bifurcated root?
   A. Mandibular central incisor
   B. Maxillary central incisor
   C. Mandibular canine
   D. Maxillary canine
4. Which cusp ridge is longer on a permanent maxillary canine?
   A. Mesial
   B. Distal
   C. They are equal in length.
   D. The maxillary canine does not have any cusp ridges.

5. The root length of the permanent mandibular canine is closest to which of the following?
   A. 14 mm
   B. 16 mm
   C. 18 mm
   D. 20 mm

For additional study resources, please visit Expert Consult.

The maxillary and mandibular canines bear a close resemblance to each other, and their functions are closely related. The four canines are placed at the "corners" of the mouth; each one is the third tooth from the median line, right and left, in the maxilla and mandible. They are commonly referred to as the *cornerstones* of the dental arches.[1] They are the longest teeth in the mouth; the crowns are usually as long as those of the maxillary central incisors, and the single roots are longer than those of any of the other teeth. The middle labial lobes have been highly developed incisally into strong, well-formed cusps. Crowns and roots are markedly convex on most surfaces. The shapes and positions of the canines contribute to the guidance of the teeth into the intercuspal position by "canine guidance."[2]

The shape of the crowns—with their single pointed cusps, their locations in the mouth, and the extra anchorage furnished by the long, strongly developed roots—makes these canines resemble those of the carnivore. This resemblance to the prehensile teeth of the carnivore gives rise to the term **canine.**

Because of the labiolingual thickness of crown and root and the anchorage in the alveolar process of the jaws, these teeth are perhaps the most stable in the mouth. The crown portions of the canines are shaped in a manner that promotes cleanliness. This self-cleansing quality, along with the efficient anchorage in the jaws, tends to preserve these teeth throughout life. When teeth are lost, the canines are usually the last to go. They are very valuable teeth considered either as units of the natural dental arches or as possible assistants in stabilizing replacements of lost teeth in prosthetic procedures.

Both maxillary and mandibular canines have another quality that must not be overlooked: the positions and forms of these teeth and their anchorage in the bone, along with the bone ridge over the labial portions of the roots, called the **canine eminence,** have a cosmetic value. They help form a foundation that ensures normal facial expression at the corners of the mouth. Loss of all of these teeth makes it extremely difficult or impossible to make replacements that restore the natural appearance of the face for any length of

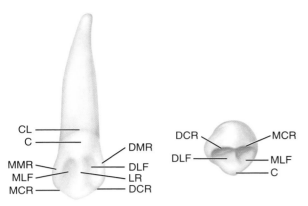

• **Fig. 8.1** Maxillary right canine, lingual and incisal aspects. *C,* Cingulum; *CL,* cervical line; *DCR,* distal cusp ridge; *DLF,* distolingual fossa; *DMR,* distal marginal ridge; *LR,* lingual ridge; *MCR,* mesial cusp ridge; *MLF,* mesiolingual fossa; *MMR,* mesial marginal ridge.

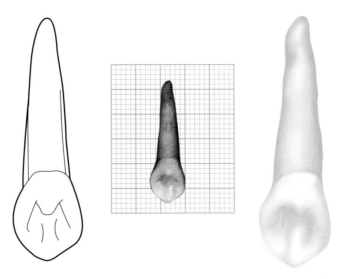

• **Fig. 8.3** Maxillary left canine, lingual aspect. (Grid = 1 sq. mm.)

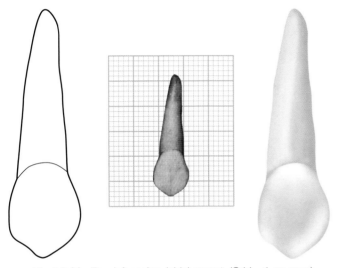

• **Fig. 8.2** Maxillary left canine, labial aspect. (Grid = 1 sq. mm.)

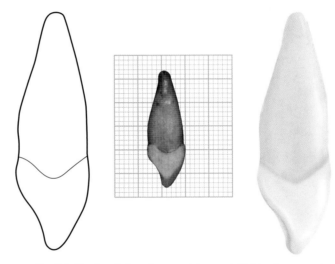

• **Fig. 8.4** Maxillary left canine, mesial aspect. (Grid = 1 sq. mm.)

time. It would therefore be difficult to place a value on the canines, and their importance is manifested by their efficiency in function, stability, and aid in maintaining natural facial expression.

In function, the canines support the incisors and premolars, since they are located between these groups. The canine crowns have some characteristics of functional form, which bears a resemblance to incisor form and also to the premolar form.

Maxillary Canine

Figs. 8.1 through 8.12 illustrate the maxillary canine in various aspects. The outline of the labial or lingual aspect of the maxillary canine is a series of curves or arcs except for the angle made by the tip of the cusp. This cusp has a mesial incisal ridge and a distal incisal ridge.

The mesial half of the crown makes contact with the lateral incisor, and the distal half contacts the first premolar. Therefore the contact areas of the maxillary canine are at different levels cervicoincisally.

From a labial view, the mesial half of the crown resembles a portion of an incisor, whereas the distal half resembles a

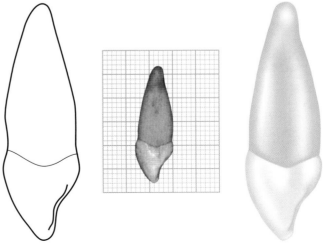

• **Fig. 8.5** Maxillary left canine, distal aspect. (Grid = 1 sq. mm.)

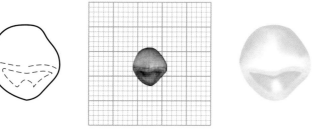

• **Fig. 8.6** Maxillary left canine, incisal aspect. (Grid = 1 sq. mm.)

portion of a premolar. This tooth seems to be a compromise in the change from anterior to posterior teeth in the dental arch.

It is apparent that the construction of this tooth has reinforcement, labiolingually, to offset directional lines of the force brought against it when in use. The incisal (incising) portion is thicker labiolingually than that of either the maxillary central or the lateral incisor.

The labiolingual measurement of the crown is about 1 mm greater than that of the maxillary central incisor (Table 8.1). The mesiodistal measurement is approximately 1 mm less.

The cingulum shows greater development than that of the central incisor.

The root of the maxillary canine is usually the longest of any root with the possible exception of that of the mandibular

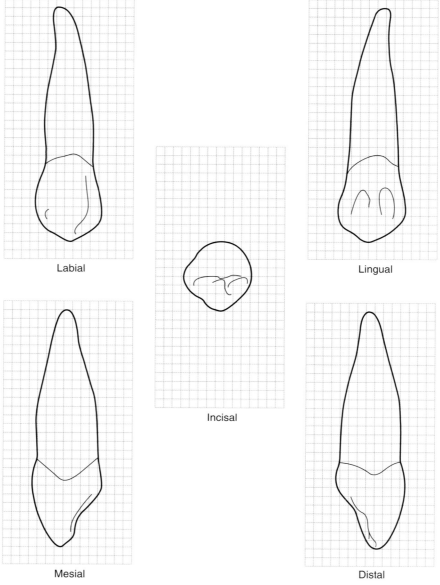

Labial

Lingual

Incisal

Mesial

Distal

• **Fig. 8.7** Maxillary right canine. Graph outlines of five aspects are shown. (Grid = 1 sq. mm.)

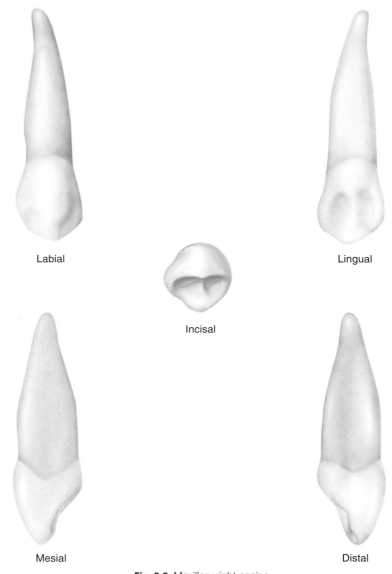

Labial

Lingual

Incisal

Mesial

Distal

• **Fig. 8.8** Maxillary right canine.

canine, which may be as long at times. The root is thick labio-lingually, with developmental depressions mesially and distally that help furnish the secure anchorage this tooth has in the maxilla. Uncommon variations are shown in Fig. 8.12.

Detailed Description of the Maxillary Canine From All Aspects

Labial Aspect

From the labial aspect, the crown and root are narrower mesiodistally than the crown and root of the maxillary central incisor. The difference is about 1 mm in most mouths. The cervical line labially is convex, with the convexity toward the root portion (see Figs. 8.2 and 8.7 through 8.9).

Mesially, the outline of the crown may be convex from the cervix to the center of the mesial contact area, or the crown may exhibit a slight concavity above the contact area from the labial aspect. The center of the contact area mesially is approximately at the junction of middle and incisal thirds of the crown.

Distally, the outline of the crown is usually concave between the cervical line and the distal contact area. The distal contact area is usually at the center of the middle third of the crown. The two levels of contact areas mesially and distally should be noted (see Fig. 5.7B and C).

Unless the crown has been worn unevenly, the cusp tip is on a line with the center of the root. The cusp has a mesial slope and a distal slope, the mesial slope being the shorter of the two. Both slopes show a tendency toward concavity before wear has taken place (see Fig. 8.9, 5 and 6). These depressions are developmental in character.

The labial surface of the crown is smooth, with no developmental lines of note except shallow depressions mesially and distally dividing the three labial lobes. The middle labial lobe shows much greater development than the other lobes. This produces a ridge on the labial surface of the crown. A line drawn over the crest of this ridge, from the cervical line to the tip of the cusp, is a curved one inclined mesially at its center. All areas mesial to the crest of this ridge exhibit convexity except for insignificant developmental lines in the enamel.

TABLE 8.2   **Mandibular Canine**

First evidence of calcification	4–5 months
Enamel completed	6–7 years
Eruption	9–10 years
Root completed	12–14 years

MEASUREMENT TABLE							
			Mesiodistal Diameter of Crown at	Labio- or Buccolingual Diameter of	Labio- or Buccolingual Diameter of Crown at		
	Cervicoincisal Length of Crown	Length of Root	Mesiodistal Diameter of Crown	of Crown at Cervix	Diameter of Crown	of Crown at Cervix	Curvature of Cervical Line, Mesial	Curvature of Cervical Line, Distal
Dimensions[a] suggested for carving technique	11.0	16.0	7.0	5.5	7.5	7.0	2.5	1.0

[a]In millimeters.

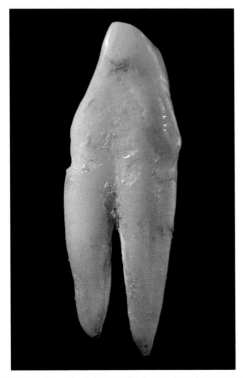

• **Fig. 8.25** Mesial view of a left mandibular canine demonstrating prominent root bifurcation.

• The cusp tip and mesial cusp ridge are more likely to be inclined in a lingual direction in the mandibular canine, with the distal cusp ridge and the contact area extension distinctly so. Note that the cusp ridges of the maxillary canine with the contact area extensions are more nearly in a straight line mesiodistally from the incisal aspect. (To view Animations 3 and 4, please go to Expert Consult.)

Pretest Answers

1. B
2. C
3. C
4. B
5. B

References

1. Kraus BS: *Dental anatomy and occlusion*, Baltimore, 1969, Williams & Wilkins.
2. Ash MM, Ramfjord SP: *Occlusion*, ed 4, Philadelphia, 1995, Saunders.

9

The Permanent Maxillary Premolars

Pretest Questions

1. Statement 1: The mesial slope of the buccal cusp of a maxillary first premolar is rather straight and shorter than the distal cusp slope. Statement 2: As a result, the buccal cusp tip is shifted mesial to a line bisecting the buccal surface of the crown.
   A. Statement 1 and 2 are true as written.
   B. Statement 1 is true while Statement 2 is false as written.
   C. Statement 1 is false while Statement 2 is true as written.
   D. Statement 1 and 2 are false as written.
2. If a maxillary premolar possesses two roots, which of the following explains their positioning?
   A. One buccal, one lingual
   B. One mesial, one distal
   C. Usually fused
   D. Maxillary premolars never possess two roots
3. A deep developmental depression exists on which of the following surfaces of the maxillary first premolar?
   A. Buccal
   B. Lingual
   C. Mesial
   D. Distal
4. What is the length of the root of the maxillary second premolar?
   A. 14 mm
   B. 15 mm
   C. 16 mm
   D. 17 mm
5. At what age does the maxillary second premolar begin eruption?
   A. 7 to 8 years
   B. 8 to 9 years
   C. 9 to 10 years
   D. 10 to 12 years

For additional study resources, please visit Expert Consult.

The maxillary premolars number four: two in the right maxilla and two in the left maxilla. They are posterior to the canines and immediately anterior to the molars.

The premolars are so named because they are anterior to the molars in the permanent dentition. In zoology, the premolars are those teeth that succeed the deciduous molars regardless of the number to be succeeded. The term **bicuspid**, which is widely used to describe human teeth, presupposes two cusps, a supposition that makes the term misleading, because mandibular premolars in the human may show a variation in the number of cusps from one to three. Among carnivores, in the study of comparative dental anatomy, premolar forms differ so greatly that a more descriptive single term than premolar is out of the question. The term **premolar** is used widely in dental anatomy, human and comparative; therefore, it will be used here. However, its use here does not suggest that the term *bicuspid* should not be used when appropriate.

The maxillary premolars are developed from the same number of lobes as anterior teeth—four. The primary difference in development is the well-formed lingual cusp, developed from the lingual lobe, which is represented by the cingulum development on incisors and canines. The middle buccal lobe on the premolars, corresponding to the middle labial lobe of the canines, remains highly developed, with the maxillary premolars resembling the canines when viewed from the buccal aspect. The buccal cusp of the maxillary first premolar, especially, is long and sharp, assisting the canine as a prehensile or tearing tooth. The mandibular first premolar assists the mandibular canine in the same manner.

The second premolars, both maxillary and mandibular, have cusps less sharp than the others, and their cusps articulate with opposing teeth when the jaws are brought together; this makes them more efficient as grinding teeth, and they function much like the molars, but to a lesser degree.

The maxillary premolar crowns are shorter than those of the maxillary canines, and the roots are also shorter. The root lengths equal those of the molars. The crowns are a little longer than those of the molars.

Because of the cusp development buccally and lingually, the marginal ridges are in a more horizontal plane and are considered part of the occlusal surface of the crown rather than part of the lingual surface, as in the case of incisors and canines.

When premolars have two roots, one is placed buccally and one lingually.

Maxillary First Premolar

Figs. 9.1 through 9.16 illustrate the maxillary first premolar from all aspects. The maxillary first premolar has two cusps, a buccal and a lingual, each being sharply defined. The buccal cusp is usually about 1 mm longer than the lingual cusp. The crown is angular, and the buccal line angles are prominent.

The crown is shorter than that of the canine by 1.5 to 2 mm on the average (Table 9.1). Although this tooth resembles the canine from the buccal aspect, it differs in that the contact areas mesially and distally are at about the same level. The root is shorter. If the buccal cusp form has not been changed by wear, the mesial slope of the cusp is longer than the distal slope. The opposite arrangement is true of the maxillary canine. In general, the first premolar is not as wide in a mesiodistal direction as the canine.

Most maxillary first premolars have two roots (see Fig. 9.10) and two pulp canals. When only one root is present, two pulp canals are usually found anyway.

The maxillary first premolar has some characteristics common to all posterior teeth. Briefly, those characteristics that differentiate posterior teeth from anterior teeth are as follows:

1. Greater relative faciolingual measurement compared with the mesiodistal measurement
2. Broader contact areas
3. Contact areas more nearly at the same level
4. Less curvature of the cervical line mesially and distally
5. Shorter crown cervico-occlusally than that of anterior teeth

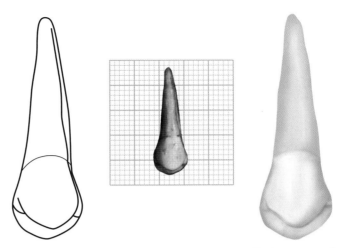

• **Fig. 9.3** Maxillary left first premolar, lingual aspect. (Grid = 1 sq. mm.)

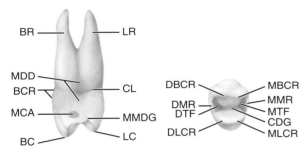

• **Fig. 9.1** Maxillary right first premolar, mesial and occlusal aspects. *BC,* Buccal cusp; *BCR,* buccal cervical ridge; *BR,* buccal root; *CDG,* central developmental groove; *CL,* cervical line; *DBCR,* distobuccal cusp ridge; *DLCR,* distolingual cusp ridge; *DMR,* distal marginal ridge; *DTF,* distal triangular fossa; *LC,* lingual cusp; *LR,* Lingual root; *MBCR,* mesiobuccal cusp ridge; *MCA,* mesial contact area; *MDD,* mesial developmental depression; *MLCR,* mesiolingual cusp ridge; *MMDG,* mesial marginal developmental groove; *MMR,* mesial marginal ridge; *MTF,* mesial triangular fossa *(shaded area).*

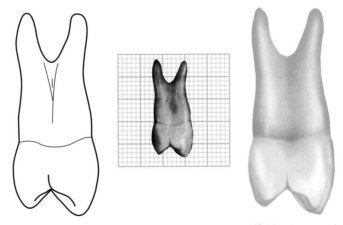

• **Fig. 9.4** Maxillary left first premolar, mesial aspect. (Grid = 1 sq. mm.)

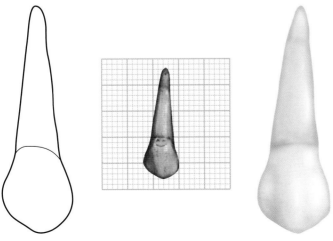

• **Fig. 9.2** Maxillary left first premolar, buccal aspect. (Grid = 1 sq. mm.)

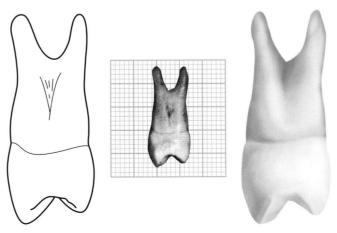

• **Fig. 9.5** Maxillary left first premolar, distal aspect. (Grid = 1 sq. mm.)

Detailed Description of the Maxillary First Premolar From All Aspects

Buccal Aspect

From the buccal aspect, the crown is roughly trapezoidal (see Fig. 4.16C). The crown exhibits little curvature at the cervical line. The

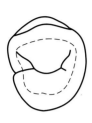 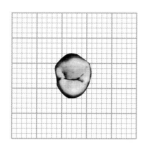 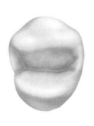

• **Fig. 9.6** Maxillary left first premolar, occlusal aspect. (Grid = 1 sq. mm.)

crest of curvature of the cervical line buccally is near the center of the root buccally (see Figs. 9.2 and 9.7 through 9.9).

The mesial outline of the crown is slightly concave from the cervical line to the mesial contact area. The contact area is represented by a relatively broad curvature, the crest of which lies immediately occlusal to the halfway point from the cervical line to the tip of the buccal cusp.

The mesial slope of the buccal cusp is rather straight and longer than the distal slope, which is shorter and more curved. This arrangement places the tip of the buccal cusp distal to a line bisecting the buccal surface of the crown. The mesial slope of the buccal cusp is sometimes notched; in other instances, a concave outline is noted at this point (see Fig. 9.9, *7, 9,* and *10*).

The distal outline of the crown below the cervical line is straighter than that of the mesial, although it may be somewhat concave as well. The distal contact area is represented by a broader curvature than is found mesially, and the crest of curvature of the contact area tends to be a little more occlusal when the tooth is

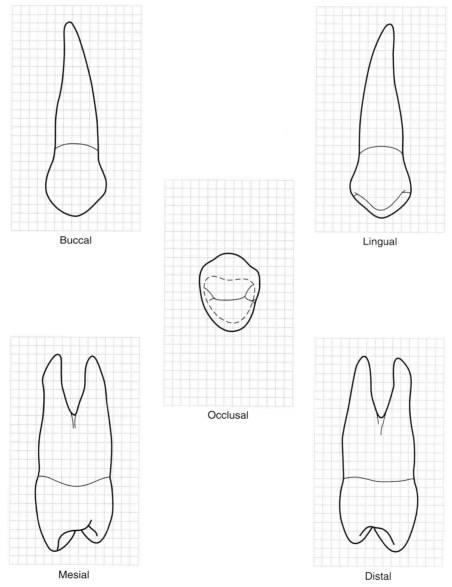

Buccal

Lingual

Occlusal

Mesial

Distal

• **Fig. 9.7** Maxillary right first premolar. Graph outlines of five aspects are shown. (Grid = 1 sq. mm.)

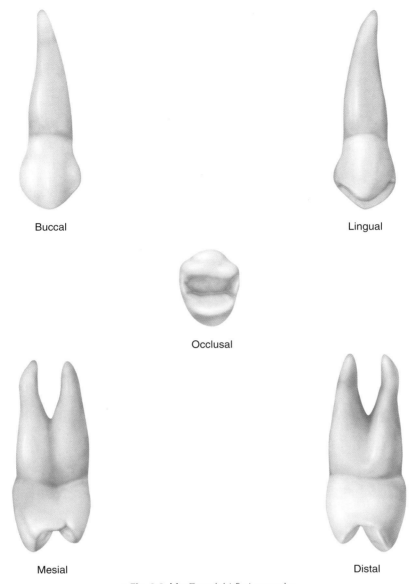

Buccal

Lingual

Occlusal

Mesial

Distal

• **Fig. 9.8** Maxillary right first premolar.

posed with its long axis vertical. Even so, the contact areas are more nearly level with each other than those found on anterior teeth.

The width of the crown of the maxillary first premolar mesiodistally is about 2 mm less at the cervix than at its width at the points of its greatest mesiodistal measurement.

The buccal cusp is long, coming to a pointed tip and resembling the canine in this respect, although contact areas in this tooth are near the same level.

The buccal surface of the crown is convex, showing strong development of the middle buccal lobe. The continuous ridge from cusp tip to cervical margin on the buccal surface of the crown is called the **buccal ridge**.

Mesial and distal to the buccal ridge, at or occlusal to the middle third, developmental depressions are usually seen that serve as demarcations between the middle buccal lobe and the mesiobuccal and distobuccal lobes. Although the latter lobes show less development, they are nevertheless prominent and serve to emphasize strong mesiobuccal and distobuccal line angles on the crown.

The roots are 3 or 4 mm shorter than those of the maxillary canine, although the outline of the buccal portion of the root form bears a close resemblance.

Lingual Aspect

From the lingual aspect, the gross outline of the maxillary first premolar is the reverse of the gross outline from the buccal aspect (see Figs. 9.3, 9.7, and 9.8).

The crown tapers toward the lingual because the lingual cusp is narrower mesiodistally than the buccal cusp. The lingual cusp is smooth and spheroidal from the cervical portion to the area near the cusp tip. The cusp tip is pointed, with mesial and distal slopes meeting at an angle of about 90 degrees.

Naturally, the spheroidal form of the lingual portion of the crown is convex at all points. Sometimes the crest of the smooth lingual portion that terminates at the point of the lingual cusp is called the **lingual ridge**.

The mesial and distal outlines of the lingual portion of the crown are convex; these outlines are continuous with the mesial

1 2 3 4 5

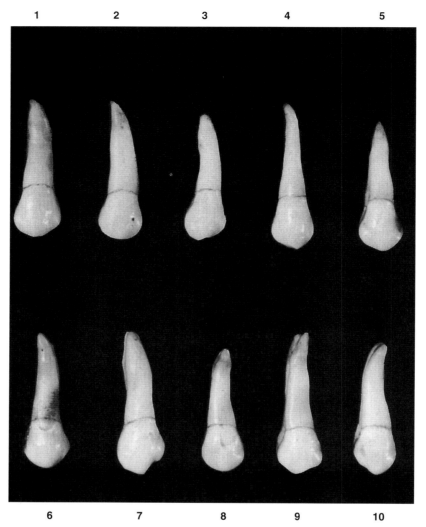

6 7 8 9 10

• **Fig. 9.9** Maxillary first premolar, buccal aspect. Ten typical specimens are shown. (To view Animations 3 and 4 for tooth #5, please go to Expert Consult.)

and distal slopes of the lingual cusp and straighten out as they join the mesial and distal sides of the lingual root at the cervical line.

The cervical line lingually is regular, with slight curvature toward the root and the crest of curvature centered on the root. Because the lingual portion of the crown is narrower than the buccal portion, it is possible to see part of the mesial and distal surfaces of crown and root from the lingual aspect, depending on the posing of the tooth and the line of vision.

Because the lingual cusp is not as long as the buccal cusp, the tips of both cusps, with their mesial and distal slopes, may be seen from the lingual aspect.

The lingual portion of the root, or the lingual portion of the lingual root if two roots are present, is smooth and convex at all points. The apex of the lingual root of a two-root specimen tends to be blunter than the buccal root apex.

Mesial Aspect

The mesial aspect of the crown of the maxillary first premolar is also roughly trapezoidal (see Figs. 9.1, 9.4, 9.7, 9.8, and 9.10). However, the longest of the uneven sides is toward the cervical portion, and the shortest is toward the occlusal portion (see Fig. 4.16E).

Another characteristic that is representative of all posterior maxillary teeth is that the tips of the cusps are well within the confines of the root trunk. (For a definition of root trunk, see Figs. 11.3 and 11.8.) In other words, the measurement from the tip of the buccal cusp to the tip of the lingual cusp is less than the buccolingual measurement of the root at its cervical portion.

Most maxillary first premolars have two roots, one buccal and one lingual; these are clearly outlined from the mesial aspect.

The cervical line may be regular in outline (see Fig. 9.10, 1) or irregular (see Fig. 9.10, 4). In either case, the curvature occlusally is less (about 1 mm on the average) than the cervical curvature on the mesial of any of the anterior teeth. The extent of the curvature of the cervical line mesially on these teeth is constant within a fraction of a millimeter and is similar to the average curvature of the mesial of all posterior teeth.

From the mesial aspect, the buccal outline of the crown curves outward below the cervical line. The crest of curvature is often located approximately at the junction of cervical and middle thirds; however, the crest of curvature may be located within the cervical third (see Fig. 9.10, 1 and 10). From the crest of curvature, the buccal outline continues as a line of less convexity to the

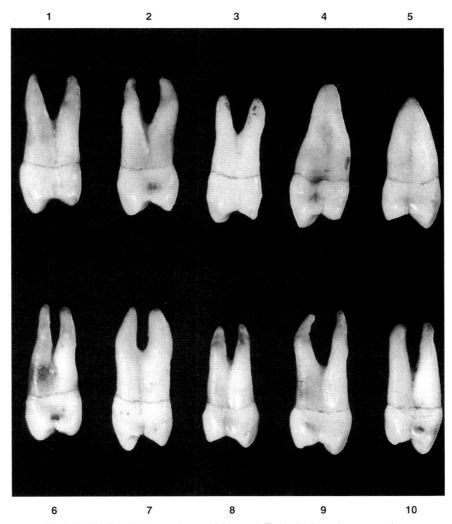

• **Fig. 9.10** Maxillary first premolar, mesial aspect. Ten typical specimens are shown.

tip of the buccal cusp, which is directly below the center of the buccal root (when two roots are present).

The lingual outline of the crown may be described as a smoothly curved line starting at the cervical line and ending at the tip of the lingual cusp. The crest of this curvature is most often near the center of the middle third. Some specimens show a more abrupt curvature at the cervical third (see Fig. 9.10, *2* and *9*).

The tip of the lingual cusp is on a line, in most cases, with the lingual border of the lingual root. The lingual cusp is always shorter than the buccal cusp, the average difference being about 1 mm. This difference, however, may be greater (see Fig. 9.10, *1, 4,* and *10*). From this aspect, it is noted that the cusps of the maxillary first premolar are long and sharp, with the mesial marginal ridge at about the level of the junction of the middle and occlusal thirds.

A distinguishing feature of this tooth is found on the mesial surface of the crown. Immediately cervical to the mesial contact area, centered on the mesial surface and bordered buccally and lingually by the mesiobuccal and mesiolingual line angles, is a marked depression called the **mesial developmental depression** (see Fig. 9.1). This mesial concavity continues apically beyond the cervical line, joins a deep developmental depression between the roots, and ends at the root bifurcation.

On single-root specimens, the concavity on the crown and root is also plainly seen, although it may not be as deeply marked. Maxillary second premolars do not have this feature (see Fig. 9.11A and B).

Another distinguishing feature of the maxillary first premolar is a well-defined developmental groove in the enamel of the mesial marginal ridge. This groove is in alignment with the developmental depression on the mesial surface of the root but is not usually connected with it. This marginal groove is continuous with the central groove of the occlusal surface of the crown, crossing the marginal ridge immediately lingual to the mesial contact area and terminating a short distance cervical to the mesial marginal ridge on the mesial surface (see Fig. 9.10, *10*).

The buccal outline of the buccal root, above the cervical line, is straight, with a tendency toward a lingual inclination. On those buccal roots having a buccal inclination above the root bifurcation, the outline may be relatively straight up to the apical portion of the buccal root or it may curve buccally at the middle third. Buccal roots may take a buccal or lingual inclination, apical to middle thirds.

The lingual outline of the lingual root is rather straight above the cervical line. It may not exhibit much curvature between the cervix and the apex. Many cases, however, show considerable curvature to

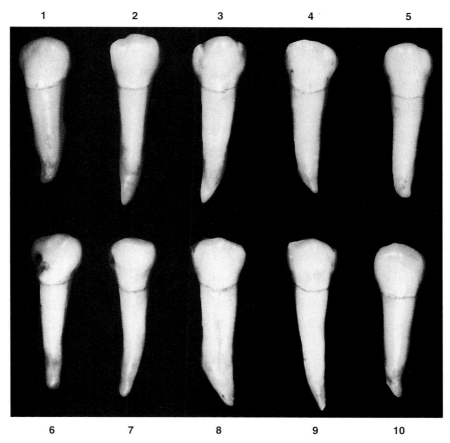

• **Fig. 10.18** Mandibular second premolar, buccal aspect. Ten typical specimens are shown. (To view Animations 3 and 4 for tooth #29, please go to Expert Consult.)

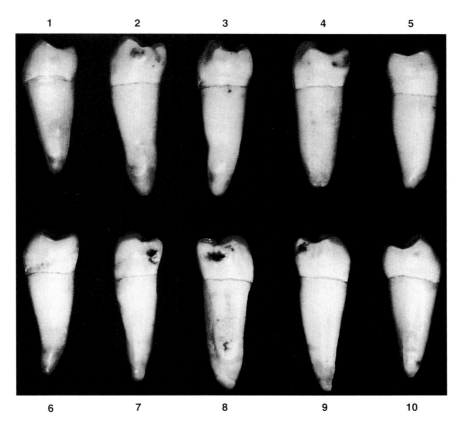

• **Fig. 10.19** Mandibular second premolar, mesial aspect. Ten typical specimens are shown.

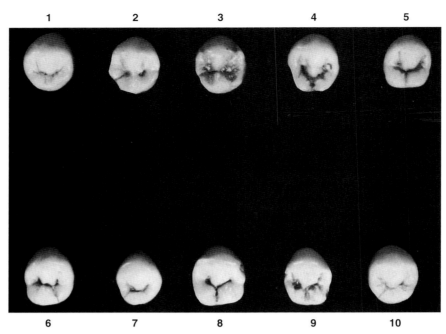

• **Fig. 10.20** Mandibular second premolar, occlusal aspect. Ten typical specimens are shown.

ends in an apex that is more blunt. In other respects, the two teeth are quite similar from this aspect.

Lingual Aspect

From the lingual aspect, the second premolar crown shows considerable variation from the crown portion of the first premolar (see Fig. 10.14). The variations are as follows:
1. The lingual lobes are developed to a greater degree, which makes the cusp or cusps (depending on the type) longer.
2. Less of the occlusal surface may be seen from this aspect. Nevertheless, because the lingual cusps are not as long as the buccal cusp, part of the buccal portion of the occlusal surface may be seen.
3. In the three-cusp type, the lingual development brings about the greatest variation between the two teeth. Mesiolingual and distolingual cusps are present, with the former being the larger and the longer one in most cases. A groove is between them, extending a very short distance on the lingual surface and usually centered over the root (see Fig. 10.20, *8*).

In the two-cusp type, the single lingual cusp development attains equal height with the three-cusp type. The two-cusp type has no groove, but it shows a developmental depression distolingually, where the lingual cusp ridge joins the distal marginal ridge (see Fig. 10.20, *2* and *3*).

The lingual surface of the crown of all mandibular second premolars is smooth and spheroidal, having a bulbous form above the constricted cervical portion.

The root is wide lingually, although not quite as wide as the buccal portion. Less difference in dimension is evident here than was found on the first premolar, so that much less convergence toward the lingual is seen.

Because in most instances the lingual portion of the crown converges little from the buccal portion, less of the mesial and distal sides of this tooth may be seen from this aspect than are seen from the lingual aspect of the first premolar.

The lingual portion of the root is smoothly convex for most of its length. Considered overall, the second premolar is the larger of the two mandibular premolars.

Mesial Aspect

From the mesial aspect (see Figs. 10.15 and 10.19), the second premolar differs from the first premolar as follows:
1. The crown and root are wider buccolingually.
2. The buccal cusp is not as nearly centered over the root trunk, and it is shorter.
3. The lingual lobe development is greater.
4. The marginal ridge is at right angles to the long axis of the tooth.
5. Less of the occlusal surface may be seen.
6. No mesiolingual developmental groove is present on the crown portion.
7. The root is longer and in most cases slightly convex on the mesial surface; however, this convexity is not always present (see Fig. 10.19, *6, 7,* and *8*).
8. The apex of the root is usually blunter on the second premolar.

Distal Aspect

The distal aspect of the mandibular second premolar is similar to the mesial aspect, except that more of the occlusal surface may be seen (see Fig. 10.16). This is possible because the distal marginal ridge is at a lower level than the mesial marginal ridge when the tooth is posed vertically. The crowns of all posterior teeth are tipped distally to the long axes of the roots, so that when the specimen tooth is held vertically, more of the occlusal surface may be seen from the distal aspect than from the mesial aspect. This is a characteristic possessed by all posterior teeth, mandibular and maxillary. The angulation of occlusal surfaces to long axes of all posterior teeth is an important observation to remember, not only in the study of individual tooth forms but also later, in the study of alignment and occlusion.

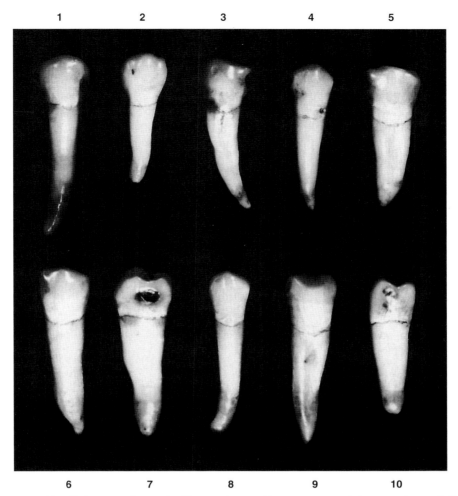

• **Fig. 10.21** Mandibular second premolar. Ten specimens with uncommon variations are shown. *1,* Root extremely long. *2,* Root dwarfed. *3,* Malformed root; developmental groove on buccal surface. *4,* Contact areas on crown high and constricted. *5,* Crown oversized; developmental groove buccally on root. *6,* Root oversized. *7,* Root malformed and of extra length. *8,* Root very long with blunt apex; extreme curvature at apical third. *9,* Crown and root oversized; developmental groove buccally on root. *10,* Crown narrow buccolingually; very little curvature buccally and lingually.

Occlusal Aspect

As mentioned earlier, two common forms of this tooth are evident. The outline form of each type shows some variation from the occlusal aspect (see Figs. 10.17 and 10.20). The two types are similar in that portion that is buccal to the mesiobuccal and distobuccal cusp ridges.

The three-cusp type appears square lingual to the buccal cusp ridges when highly developed (see Fig. 10.20, *8*). The round, or two-cusp, type appears round lingual to the buccal cusp ridges (see Fig. 10.20, *3*).

The square type (see Fig. 10.20, *8*) has three cusps that are distinct; the buccal cusp is the largest, the mesiolingual cusp is next, and the distolingual cusp is the smallest.

Each cusp has well-formed triangular ridges separated by deep developmental grooves. These grooves converge in a **central pit** and form a Y shape on the occlusal surface. The central pit is located midway between the buccal cusp ridge and the lingual margin of the occlusal surface and slightly distal to the central point between the mesial and distal marginal ridges.

Starting at the central pit, the *mesial developmental groove* travels in a mesiobuccal direction and ends in the **mesial triangular fossa** just distal to the mesial marginal ridge. The distal developmental groove travels in a distobuccal direction, is somewhat shorter than the mesial groove, and ends in the distal triangular fossa mesial to the distal marginal side. The lingual developmental groove extends lingually between the two lingual cusps and ends on the lingual surface of the crown just below the convergence of the lingual cusp ridges. The mesiolingual cusp is wider mesiodistally than the distolingual cusp. This arrangement places the lingual developmental groove distal to center on the crown.

Supplemental grooves and depressions are often seen, radiating from the developmental grooves. Occasionally, a groove crosses one or both of the marginal ridges. On a tooth of this type, the point angles are distinct. Developmental grooves are often deep.

Fig. 10.20, *8* is representative. Variations of this development may be seen in Fig. 10.20, *4, 5, 6,* and *9.*

TABLE 10.2	**Mandibular Second Premolar**

First evidence of calcification	2¼–2½ years
Enamel completed	6–7 years
Eruption	11–12 years
Root completed	13–14 years

MEASUREMENT TABLE							
	Cervico-Occlusal Length of Crown	Length of Root	Mesiodistal Diameter of Crown	Mesiodistal Diameter of Crown at Cervix	Labio- or Buccolingual Diameter of Crown	Labio- or Buccolingual Diameter of Crown at Cervix	Curvature of Cervical Line—Mesial	Curvature of Cervical Line—Distal
Dimensions[a] suggested for carving technique	8.0	14.5	7.0	5.0	8.0	7.0	1.0	0.0

[a]In millimeters.

The round or two-cusp type (see Fig. 10.20, *3*) differs considerably from the three-cusp type when viewed from the occlusal aspect. It is a true typal form of the two-cusp type. Variations may be seen in Fig. 10.20, *1*, *2*, *7*, and *10*.

The occlusal characteristics of the two-cusp type are as follows:

1. The outline of the crown is rounded lingual to the buccal cusp ridges.
2. Some lingual convergence of mesial and distal sides occurs, although no more than is found in some variations of the square type.
3. The mesiolingual and distolingual line angles are rounded.
4. One well-developed lingual cusp is directly opposite the buccal cusp in a lingual direction.

A **central developmental groove** on the occlusal surface travels in a mesiodistal direction. This groove may be straight (see Fig. 10.20, *3*), but it is most often crescent shaped (see Fig. 10.20, *1*, *7*, and *10*). The central groove has its terminals centered in *mesial* and *distal fossae*, which are roughly circular depressions having supplemental grooves and depressions radiating from the central groove and its terminals. The enamel surface inside these fossae and around their peripheries is very irregular, acting as a contrast to the smoothness of cusp ridges, marginal ridges, and the transverse ridge from the buccal cusp to the lingual cusp.

Some of these teeth show **mesial** and **distal developmental pits** centered in the mesial and distal fossae instead of an unbroken central groove (see Fig. 10.20, *2*).

Although photographs do not demonstrate it very well, most of these two-cusp specimens show a developmental depression crossing the distolingual cusp ridge. (To view Animations 3 and 4, please go to Expert Consult.)

Pretest Answers

1. B
2. A
3. D
4. D
5. A

Bibliography

Carlsen O: Human lower premolars: macro-morphologic observations on the ontogenesis of the root complex, *Scand J Dent Res* 78:5, 1970.

Kraus B, Purr ML: Lower first premolar: a definition of discrete morphologic traits, *J Dent Res* 32:554, 1953.

Ludwig PJ: The mandibular second premolars: morphologic variation and inheritance, *J Dent Res* 36:263, 1957.

Osborn JR, editor: *Dental anatomy and embryology*, Oxford, 1981, Blackwell Scientific Publications.

Renner RP: *An introduction to dental anatomy and esthetics*, Chicago, 1985, Quintessence.

Schumacher G-H: *Odontographie: Eine Oberflächenenanatomie der Zähne*, Leipzig, 1983, JM Barth.

11

The Permanent Maxillary Molars

1. Correctly define and pronounce the new terms as emphasized in the bold type.
2. Correctly label the anatomic landmarks of permanent maxillary first, second, and third molars.
3. Discuss the grid diagrams of the permanent maxillary first, second, and third molars and be able to correctly draw the graph outlines of each tooth from all views. Note: Being able to model correct tooth contours is fundamental to learning. Drawing, waxing, and/or carving the teeth are good ways to practice this.
4. Discuss common anatomic variations seen in each tooth type.
5. List similarities and differences between permanent maxillary first, second, and third molars.

Pretest Questions

1. Which cusp of the maxillary first molar is the largest and most well formed?
   A. Mesiobuccal
   B. Mesiolingual
   C. Distolingual
   D. Distobuccal
2. Calcification of the permanent maxillary first molar begins at what age?
   A. At birth
   B. 6 months
   C. 1 year
   D. 2 years
3. Calcification of the permanent maxillary second molar begins at what age?
   A. At birth
   B. 1.5 years
   C. 2.5 years
   D. 3.5 years
4. Which of the following teeth is least likely to have roots that are fused together to act as one large, tapered root?
   A. Maxillary first molar
   B. Maxillary second molar
   C. Maxillary third molar
   D. All are equally likely to have fused roots
5. The oblique ridge found on a maxillary first molar is formed by the union of which of the following structures?
   A. Triangular ridge of the mesiobuccal cusp and the triangular ridge of the distolingual cusp
   B. Triangular ridge of the mesiolingual cusp and the triangular ridge of the distobuccal cusp
   C. Distal cusp ridge of the mesiobuccal cusp and the triangular ridge of the distolingual cusp
   D. Distal cusp ridge of the mesiolingual cusp and the triangular ridge of the distobuccal cusp

For additional study resources, please visit Expert Consult.

The maxillary molars differ in design from any of the teeth previously described. These teeth assist the mandibular molars in performing the major portion of the work in the mastication and comminution of food. They are the largest and strongest maxillary teeth, by virtue both of their bulk and of their anchorage in the jaws. Although the crowns on the molars may be somewhat shorter than those on the premolars, their dimensions are greater in every respect. The root portion may be no longer than that of the premolars, but instead of one root or a bifurcated root, the maxillary molar root is broader at the base in all directions and is trifurcated into three well-developed prongs that are actually three full-size roots emanating from a common broad base above the crown.

Generally speaking, the maxillary molars have large crowns with four well-formed cusps. They have three roots, two buccal and one lingual. The lingual root is the largest. The crowns have two buccal cusps and two lingual cusps. The outlines and curvatures of all the maxillary molars are similar. Developmental variations will be set forth under descriptions of the separate molars.

Before a detailed description of the maxillary first molar, some aspects are presented that are applicable to all first molars, mandibular and maxillary.

The permanent first molars usually appear in the oral cavity when the child is 6 years old. The mandibular molars precede the maxillary molars. The first permanent molar (maxillary or mandibular) erupts posterior to the second deciduous molar, taking up a position in contact with it. Therefore the first molar is not a succedaneous tooth because it has no predecessor. The deciduous teeth are all still in position and functioning when the first molar takes its place. Because the development of the bones of the face is downward and forward, sufficient space has been created normally at age 6 years for the accommodation of this tooth.

The normal location of the first permanent molar is at the center of the fully developed adult jaw anteroposteriorly. As a consequence of the significance of their positions and the circumstances surrounding their eruption, the first molars may also be considered cornerstones of the dental arches. A full realization of the significance of these teeth as units in the arches and their function and positions relative to the other teeth will be gained when an opportunity comes to study the arrangement of the teeth with their occlusion and the temporomandibular articulation of the jaws. Subsequent chapters cover those phases. The mandibular molars are described in Chapter 12.

Maxillary First Molar

Figs. 11.1 through 11.18 illustrate the maxillary first molar from all aspects. The crown of this tooth is wider buccolingually than mesiodistally. Usually the extra dimension buccolingually is about 1 mm (Table 11.1). This, however, varies in individuals (see Fig. 11.17, *1, 5, 7,* and *9*). From the occlusal aspect, the inequality of the measurements in the two directions appears slight. Although the crown is relatively short, it is broad both

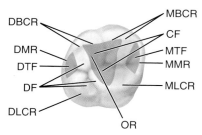

• **Fig. 11.1** Maxillary right first molar, occlusal aspect. *CF*, Central fossa *(shaded area); DBCR*, distobuccal cusp ridge; *DF*, distal fossa; *DLCR*, distolingual cusp ridge; *DMR*, distal marginal ridge; *DTF*, distal triangular fossa *(shaded area); MBCR*, Mesiobuccal cusp ridge; *MLCR*, mesiolingual cusp ridge; *MMR*, mesial marginal ridge; *MTF*, mesial triangular fossa *(shaded area); OR*, oblique ridge.

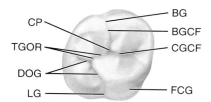

• **Fig. 11.2** Maxillary right first molar, occlusal aspect, developmental grooves. *BG*, Buccal groove; *BGCF*, buccal groove of central fossa; *CGCF*, central groove of central fossa; *CP*, central pit; *DOG*, distal oblique groove; *FCG*, fifth cusp groove; *LG*, lingual groove; *TGOR*, transverse groove of oblique ridge.

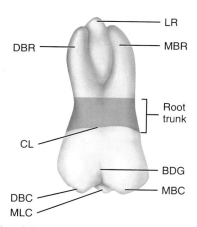

• **Fig. 11.3** Maxillary right first molar, buccal aspect. *BDG*, Buccal developmental groove; *CL*, cervical line; *DBC*, distobuccal cusp; *DBR*, distobuccal root; *LR*, Lingual root; *MBC*, mesiobuccal cusp; *MBR*, mesiobuccal root; *MLC*, mesiolingual cusp.

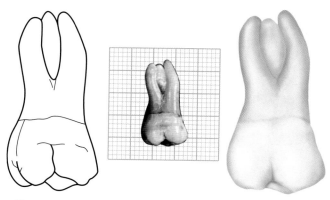

• **Fig. 11.4** Maxillary right first molar, buccal aspect. (Grid = 1 sq. mm.)

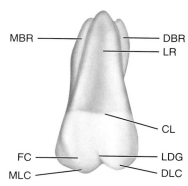

• **Fig. 11.5** Maxillary right first molar, lingual aspect. *CL*, Cervical line; *DBR*, Distobuccal root; *DLC*, distolingual cusp; *FC*, fifth cusp; *LDG*, lingual developmental groove; *LR*, lingual root; *MBR*, mesiobuccal root; *MLC*, mesiolingual cusp. (Grid = 1 sq. mm.)

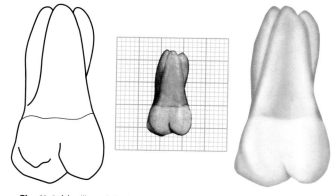

• **Fig. 11.6** Maxillary right first molar, lingual aspect. (Grid = 1 sq. mm.)

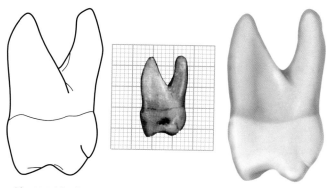

• **Fig. 11.7** Maxillary right first molar, mesial aspect. (Grid = 1 sq. mm.)

mesiodistally and buccolingually, which gives the occlusal surface its generous dimensions.

The maxillary first molar is normally the largest tooth in the maxillary arch. It has four well-developed functioning cusps and one supplemental cusp of little practical use. The four large cusps of most physiological significance are the mesiobuccal, the distobuccal, the mesiolingual, and the distolingual. A supplemental cusp is called the **cusp** or **tubercle of Carabelli.** This morphological trait

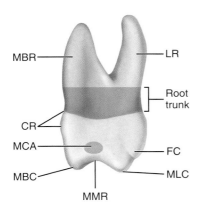

• **Fig. 11.8** Maxillary right first molar, mesial aspect. *CR,* Cervical ridge; *FC,* fifth cusp; *LR,* Lingual root; *MBC,* mesiobuccal ridge; *MBR,* mesiobuccal root; *MCA,* mesial contact area; *MLC,* mesiolingual cusp; *MMR,* mesial marginal ridge.

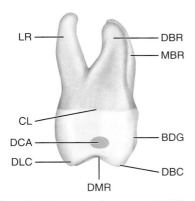

• **Fig. 11.9** Maxillary right first molar, distal aspect. *BDG,* Buccal developmental groove; *CL,* cervical line; *DBC,* distobuccal cusp; *DBR,* distobuccal root; *DCA,* distal contact area; *DLC,* distolingual cusp; *DMR,* distal marginal ridge; *LR,* lingual root; *MBR,* mesiobuccal root.

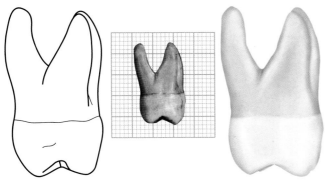

• **Fig. 11.10** Maxillary right first molar, distal aspect. (Grid = 1 sq. mm.)

can take the form of a well-developed fifth cusp, or it can grade down to a series of grooves, depressions, or pits on the mesial portion of the lingual surface. This trait has been used to distinguish populations.

This supplemental cusp is found lingual to the mesiolingual cusp, which is the largest of the well-developed cusps. Usually, a developmental groove is found, leaving a record of cusp development, unless it has been erased by frictional wear. The fifth cusp or a developmental trace at its usual site serves to identify the maxillary first molar. A specimen of this tooth showing no trace of its typical characteristic would be rare.

The three **roots** of generous proportions are the mesiobuccal, distobuccal, and lingual. These roots are well separated and well developed, and their placement gives this tooth maximum anchorage against forces that would tend to unseat it. The roots have their greatest spread parallel to the line of greatest force brought to bear against the crown diagonally in a buccolingual direction. The lingual root is the longest root. It is tapered and smoothly rounded. The mesiobuccal root is not as long, but it is broader buccolingually and shaped (in cross section) so that its resistance to torsion is greater than that of the lingual root. The distobuccal root is the smallest of the three and smoothly rounded.

The development of maxillary first molars rarely deviates from the accepted normal. Ten specimens with uncommon variations are shown in Fig. 11.18.

Detailed Description of the Maxillary First Molar From All Aspects

Buccal Aspect

The crown is roughly trapezoidal, with cervical and occlusal outlines representing the uneven sides (see Figs. 11.4 and 11.13–11.15). The cervical line is the shorter of the uneven sides (see Fig. 4.16D).

When the buccal aspect of this tooth is viewed with the line of vision at right angles to the buccal developmental groove of

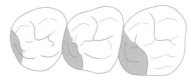

• **Fig. 11.11** Maxillary molar primary cusp triangle. The distolingual lobe, represented by shaded areas, becomes progressively smaller on maxillary molars, starting with the first molar, which presents the greatest development of the lobe. The plain areas, roughly triangular in outline, represent the *maxillary molar primary cusp triangles.*

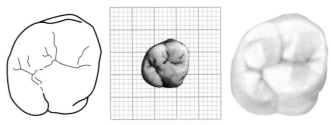

• **Fig. 11.12** Maxillary right first molar, occlusal aspect. (Grid = 1 sq. mm.). (To view Animations 3 and 4 for tooth #3, please go to Expert Consult.)

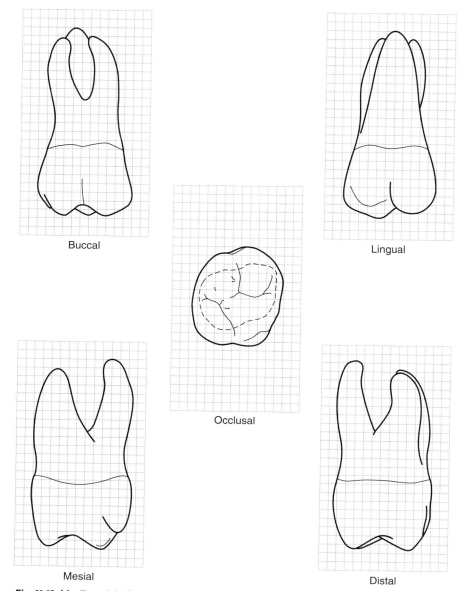

Buccal

Lingual

Occlusal

Mesial

Distal

• **Fig. 11.13** Maxillary right first molar. Graph outlines of five aspects are shown. (Grid = 1 sq. mm.)

the crown, the distal side of the crown can be seen in perspective, which is possible because of the obtuse character of the distobuccal line angle (see the section "Occlusal Aspect"). Parts of four cusps are seen: the mesiobuccal, distobuccal, mesiolingual, and distolingual.

The mesiobuccal cusp is broader than the distobuccal cusp, and its mesial slope meets its distal slope at an obtuse angle. The mesial slope of the distobuccal cusp meets its distal slope at approximately a right angle. The distobuccal cusp is therefore sharper than the mesiobuccal cusp, and it is at least as long and often longer (see Fig. 11.15, *4, 6, 7, 8,* and *9*).

The buccal developmental groove that divides the two buccal cusps is approximately equidistant between the mesiobuccal and distolingual line angles. The groove slants occlusoapically in a line of direction parallel to the long axis of the distobuccal root. It terminates at a point approximately half the distance from its origin occlusally to the cervical line of the crown. Although the groove is not deep at any point, it becomes more

shallow toward its termination, gradually fading out. Lateral to its terminus is a dip in the enamel of the crown that is developmental in character and extends for some distance mesially and distally.

The cervical line of the crown does not have much curvature from mesial to distal; however, it is not as smooth and regular as that found on some of the other teeth. The line is generally convex with the convexity toward the roots.

The mesial outline of the crown from this aspect follows a nearly straight path downward and mesially, curving occlusally as it reaches the crest of contour of the mesial surface, which is the contact area. This crest is approximately two-thirds the distance from the cervical line to the tip of the mesiobuccal cusp. The mesial outline continues downward and distally and becomes congruent with the outline of the mesial slope of the mesiobuccal cusp.

The distal outline of the crown is convex; the distal surface is spheroidal. The crest of curvature on the distal side of the crown is on the mesial surface of the maxillary first molar. This concavity may be continued to the mesial surface of the root trunk at its cervical third.

The mesiobuccal root is broad and flattened on its mesial surface; this flattened surface often exhibits smooth flutings for part of its length. The width of this root near the crown from the buccal surface to the point of bifurcation on the root trunk is approximately two-thirds of the crown measurement buccolingually at the cervical line. The buccal outline of the root extends upward and outward from the crown, ending at the blunt apex. The greatest projection on this root is usually buccal to the greatest projection of the crown. The lingual outline of the root is relatively straight from the bluntly rounded apex down to the bifurcation with the lingual root.

The level of the bifurcation is a little closer to the cervical line than is found between the roots buccally. A smooth depression congruent with the bifurcation extends occlusally and lingually almost to the cervical line directly above the mesiolingual line angle of the crown.

The lingual root is longer than the mesial root but is narrower from this aspect. It is banana-shaped, extending lingually with its convex outline to the lingual and its concave outline to the buccal. At its middle and apical thirds, it is outside of the confines of the greatest crown projection. Although its apex is rounded, the root appears more pointed toward the end than the mesiobuccal root.

Distal Aspect

The gross outline of the distal aspect is similar to that of the mesial aspect (see Figs. 11.9, 11.10, 11.13, and 11.14). Certain variations must be noted when the tooth is viewed from the distal aspect.

Because of the tendency of the crown to taper distally on the buccal surface, most of the buccal surface of the crown may be seen in perspective from the distal aspect. This is because the buccolingual measurement of the crown mesially is greater than the same measurement distally. All the decrease in measurement distally is a result of the slant of the buccal side of the crown.

The distal marginal ridge dips sharply in a cervical direction, exposing triangular ridges on the distal portion of the occlusal surface of the crown.

The cervical line is almost straight across from buccal to lingual. Occasionally, it curves apically 0.5 mm or so.

The distal surface of the crown is generally convex, with a smoothly rounded surface except for a small area near the distobuccal root at the cervical third. This concavity continues on to the distal surface of the distobuccal root, from the cervical line to the area of the root that is on a level with bifurcation separating the distobuccal and lingual roots.

The distobuccal root is narrower at its base than either of the others. An outline of this root, when the tooth is viewed from the distal aspect, starts buccally at a point immediately above the distobuccal cusp, follows a concave path inward for a short distance, then turns outward in a buccal direction, completing a graceful convex arc from the concavity to the rounded apex. This line lies entirely within the confines of the outline of the mesiobuccal root. The lingual outline of the root from the apex to the bifurcation is slightly concave. No concavity is evident between the bifurcation of the roots and the cervical line. However, the surface at this point on the root trunk has a tendency toward convexity.

The bifurcation here is more apical than either of the other two areas on this tooth. The area from cervical line to bifurcation is 5 mm or more in extent.

Occlusal Aspect

From the occlusal aspect, the maxillary first molar is somewhat rhomboidal. An outline following the four major cusp ridges and the marginal ridges is especially so (see Figs. 11.1, 11.2, 11.12–11.14, and 11.17).

A measurement of the crown buccolingually and mesial to the buccal and lingual grooves is greater than the measurement on the portion of the crown that is distal to these developmental grooves. Also, a measurement of the crown immediately lingual to contact areas mesiodistally is greater than the measurement immediately buccal to the contact areas. Thus, it is apparent that the maxillary first molar crown is wider mesially than distally and wider lingually than buccally.

The four major cusps are well developed, with the small minor, or fifth, cusp appearing on the lingual surface of the mesiolingual cusp near the mesiolingual line angle of the crown. The fifth cusp may be indistinct, or all the cusp form may be absent. At this site, however, traces of developmental lines are nearly always present in the enamel.

The mesiolingual cusp is the largest cusp; it is followed in size by the mesiobuccal, distolingual, distobuccal, and fifth cusps.

If reduced to a geometric schematic figure, the occlusal aspect of this molar locates the various angles of the rhomboidal figure as follows: acute angles, mesiobuccal and distolingual; and obtuse angles, mesiolingual and distobuccal.

An analysis of the design of the occlusal surfaces of maxillary molars may be summarized here. Developmentally, only three major cusps can be considered as primary, the mesiolingual cusp and the two buccal cusps. The distolingual cusp is common to all the maxillary molars; any other additional one, such as the cusp of Carabelli on first molars, must be regarded as secondary.

The triangular arrangement of cusps is reflected in the outline of the root trunks of maxillary molars when the teeth are sectioned in those areas (see Root Sections in Chapter 13). The distolingual cusp becomes progressively smaller on second and third maxillary molars, often disappearing as a major cusp (see Fig. 11.11). Thus the triangular arrangement of the three important molar cusps is called the **maxillary molar primary cusp triangle.** The characteristic triangular figure, made by tracing the cusp outlines of these cusps, the mesial marginal ridge, and the oblique ridge of the occlusal surface, is representative of all maxillary molars.

The **occlusal surface,** or **occlusal table** as it is sometimes termed, of the maxillary first molar is within the confines of the cusp ridges and marginal ridges. The morphological features are now considered.

There are two major fossae and two minor fossae. The major fossae are the **central fossa,** which is roughly triangular and mesial to the oblique ridge, and the **distal fossa,** which is roughly linear and distal to the oblique ridge.

The two minor fossae are the **mesial triangular fossa,** immediately distal to the mesial marginal ridge, and the **distal triangular fossa,** immediately mesial to the distal marginal ridge (see Fig. 11.1).

The **oblique ridge** is a ridge that crosses the occlusal surface obliquely. The union of the triangular ridge of the distobuccal cusp and the distal ridge of the mesiolingual cusp forms it. This ridge is reduced in height in the center of the occlusal surface, being about on a level with the marginal ridges of the occlusal surface. Sometimes it is crossed by a developmental groove that partially joins the two major fossae by means of its shallow sulcate groove.

The **mesial marginal ridge** and the **distal marginal ridge** are irregular ridges confluent with the mesial and distal cusp ridges of the mesial and distal major cusps.

The *central fossa* of the occlusal surface is a concave area bound by the distal slope of the mesiobuccal cusp, the mesial slope of the distobuccal cusp, the crest of the oblique ridge, and the crests of the two triangular ridges of the mesiobuccal and mesiolingual cusps. The central fossa has connecting sulci within its boundaries, with developmental grooves at the deepest portions of these sulci (sulcate grooves). In addition, it contains supplemental grooves, short grooves that are disconnected, and also the central developmental pit. A worn specimen may show developmental or sulcate grooves only.

In the center of the central fossa, the central developmental pit has sulcate developmental grooves radiating from it at obtuse angles to each other. This pit is located in the approximate center of that portion of the occlusal surface that is circumscribed by cusp ridges and marginal ridges (see Fig. 11.1). From this pit the **buccal developmental groove** radiates buccally at the bottom of the buccal sulcus of the central fossa, continuing on to the buccal surface of the crown between the buccal cusps.

Starting again at the central pit, the **central developmental groove** is seen to progress in a mesial direction at an obtuse angle to the buccal sulcate groove. The central groove at the bottom of the sulcus of the central fossa usually terminates at the apex of the *mesial triangular fossa.* Here it is joined by short, supplemental grooves that radiate from its terminus into the triangular fossa. These supplemental grooves often appear as branches of the central groove. Occasionally, one or more supplemental grooves cross the mesial marginal ridge of the crown.

The *mesial triangular fossa* is rather indistinct in outline, but it is generally triangular in shape, with its base at the mesial marginal ridge and its apex at the point where the supplemental grooves join the central groove.

An additional short developmental groove radiates from the central pit of the central fossa at an obtuse angulation to the buccal and central developmental grooves. Usually, it is considered a projection of one of these, because it is very short and usually fades out before reaching the crest of the oblique ridge. When it crosses the oblique ridge transversely, however, as it sometimes does, joining the central and distal fossae with a shallow groove, it is called the **transverse groove of the oblique ridge** (see Fig. 11.17, *3, 4,* and *5*).

The *distal fossa* of the maxillary first molar is roughly linear in form and is located immediately distal to the oblique ridge. An irregular developmental groove traverses its deepest portion. This developmental groove is called the **distal oblique groove.** It connects with the **lingual developmental groove** at the junction of the cusp ridges of the mesiolingual and distolingual cusps. These two grooves travel in the same oblique direction to the terminus of the lingual groove, which is centered below the lingual root at the approximate center of the crown lingually (see Fig. 11.5, *LDG*). If the fifth cusp development is distinct, a developmental groove outlining it joins the lingual groove near its terminus. Any part of the developmental groove that outlines a fifth cusp is called the **fifth cusp groove.**

The distal oblique groove in most cases shows several supplemental grooves. Two terminal branches usually appear, forming two sides of the triangular depression immediately mesial to the distal marginal ridge. These two sides, in combination with the slope mesial to the distal marginal ridge, form the distal triangular fossa. The distal outline of the distal marginal ridge of the crown shows a slight concavity.

The distolingual cusp is smooth and rounded from the occlusal aspect, and an outline of it, from the distal concavity of the distal marginal ridge to the lingual groove of the crown, describes an arch of an ellipse.

The lingual outline of the distolingual cusp is straight with the lingual outline of the fifth cusp, unless the fifth cusp is unusually large. In the latter case the lingual outline of the fifth cusp is more prominent lingually (see Fig. 11.17, *9*). The cusp ridge of the distolingual cusp usually extends lingually farther than the cusp ridge of the mesiolingual cusp.

Maxillary Second Molar

Figs. 11.19 through 11.27 illustrate the maxillary second molar from all aspects. The maxillary second molar supplements the first molar in function. In describing this tooth, direct comparisons are made with the first molar both in form and in development.

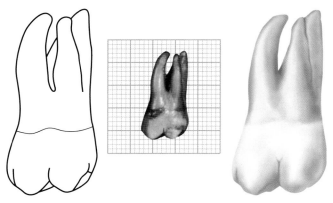

• **Fig. 11.19** Maxillary left second molar, buccal aspect. (Grid = 1 sq. mm.)

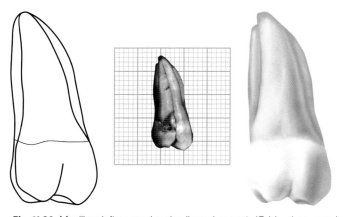

• **Fig. 11.20** Maxillary left second molar, lingual aspect. (Grid = 1 sq. mm.)

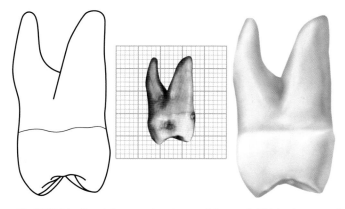

• **Fig. 11.21** Maxillary left second molar, mesial aspect. (Grid = 1 sq. mm.)

TABLE 11.3	Maxillary Third Molar

First evidence of calcification	7–9 years
Enamel completed	12–16 years
Eruption	17–21 years
Root completed	18–25 years

MEASUREMENT TABLE

	Cervico-occlusal Length of Crown	Length of Root	Mesiodistal Diameter of Crown	Mesiodistal Diameter of Crown at Cervix	Labio- or Buccolingual Diameter of Crown	Labio- or Buccolingual Diameter of Crown at Cervix	Curvature of Cervical Line—Mesial	Curvature of Cervical Line—Distal
Dimensions[a] suggested for carving technique	6.5	11.0	8.5	6.5	10.0	9.5	1.0	0.0

[a]In millimeters.

The occlusal aspect of this tooth usually presents many supplemental grooves and many accidental grooves unless the tooth is very much worn.

The third molar may show four distinct cusps. This type may have a strong oblique ridge, a central fossa and a distal fossa, with a lingual developmental groove similar to that of the rhomboidal type of second molar. In most instances, the crown converges more lingually from the buccal areas than in the second molar, losing its rhomboidal outline. This is not always true, however (compare *1* and *3* in Fig. 11.35).

Pretest Answers

1. B
2. A
3. C
4. A
5. D

Bibliography

Alexandersen V: Mandibular third molar: the root complex. II. Morphogenetic considerations, *Tandlægebladet* 66(53), 1985.

Ash MM: *Wheeler's atlas of tooth form*, ed 5, Philadelphia, 1984, Saunders.

Black GV: *Descriptive anatomy of the human teeth*, ed 4, Philadelphia, 1897, S.S. White Dental Manufacturing.

Carabelli G: *Anatomie des Mundes*, Vienna, 1842, Braumuller and Seidel.

Carbonell VM: The tubercle of Carabelli in the Kish dentition. Mesopotamia, 3000 BC, *J Dent Res* 39:124, 1960.

Carlsen O: *Dental morphology*, Copenhagen, 1987, Munksgaard.

Diamond M: *Dental anatomy*, New York, 1929, Macmillan.

Hopewell-Smith A: *An introduction to dental anatomy and physiology*, Philadelphia, 1913, Lea & Febiger.

Kraus BS: Carabelli's anomaly of the maxillary molar teeth, *Am J Hum Genet* 3:348, 1951.

Kraus BS, Jordan RE, Abrams L: *Dental anatomy and occlusion*, Baltimore, 1969, Williams & Wilkins.

Tomes CS: *A manual of dental anatomy*, London, 1894, Churchill.

Woelfel JB, Scheid RC: *Dental anatomy: its relevance to dentistry*, Baltimore, 1997, Williams & Wilkins.

12

The Permanent Mandibular Molars

LEARNING OBJECTIVES

1. Correctly define and pronounce the new terms as emphasized in the bold type.
2. Correctly label the anatomic landmarks of permanent mandibular first, second, and third molars.
3. Discuss the grid diagrams of the permanent mandibular first, second, and third molars and be able to correctly draw the graph outlines of each tooth from all views. Note: Being able to model correct tooth contours is fundamental to learning. Drawing, waxing, and/or carving the teeth are good ways to practice this.
4. Discuss common anatomic variations seen in each tooth type.
5. List similarities and differences between permanent mandibular first, second, and third molars.

Pretest Questions

1. At what age is calcification of the permanent mandibular first molar first evident?
   A. At birth
   B. 6 to 9 months
   C. 1 year
   D. 2 years
2. From the occlusal view, which of the following cusps of the permanent mandibular second molar is largest?
   A. Mesiobuccal
   B. Mesiolingual
   C. Distolingual
   D. All are about the same size
3. Statement 1: From the mesial view, all permanent mandibular posterior teeth resemble a rhombus. Statement 2: In relation to the root axis, the crown of all mandibular posterior teeth is tilted toward the buccal.
   A. Statement 1 and 2 are true as written.
   B. Statement 1 is true while Statement 2 is false as written.
   C. Statement 1 is false while Statement 2 is true as written.
   D. Statement 1 and 2 are false as written.
4. At what age is calcification of the permanent mandibular second molar first evident?
   A. At birth
   B. 6 to 9 months
   C. 1 year
   D. 2 to 3 years
5. Statement 1: There is often times not enough space in the mandibular arch for the third molars to erupt. Statement 2: As a result, partial eruption of the mandibular third molar can lead to both periodontal defects or root resorption at the distal of the second molar.
   A. Statement 1 and 2 are true as written.
   B. Statement 1 is true while Statement 2 is false as written.
   C. Statement 1 is false while Statement 2 is true as written.
   D. Statement 1 and 2 are false as written.

For additional study resources, please visit Expert Consult.

The mandibular molars are larger than any other mandibular teeth. They are three in number on each side of the mandible: the first, second, and third mandibular molars. They resemble each other in functional form, although comparison of one with another shows variations in the number of cusps and some variation in size, occlusal design, and the relative lengths and positions of the roots.

The crown outlines exhibit similarities of outline from all aspects, and each mandibular molar has two roots, one mesial and one distal. Third molars and some second molars may show a fusion of these roots. All mandibular molars have crowns that are roughly quadrilateral, being somewhat longer mesiodistally than buccolingually. Maxillary molar crowns have their widest measurement buccolingually.

The mandibular molars perform the major portion of the work of the lower jaw in mastication and in the comminution of food. They are the largest and strongest mandibular teeth, both because of their bulk and because of their anchorage.

The crowns of the molars are shorter cervico-occlusally than those of the teeth anterior to them, but their dimensions are greater in every other respect. The root portions are not as long as those of some of the other mandibular teeth, but the combined measurements of the multiple roots, with their broad bifurcated root trunks, result in superior anchorage and greater efficiency.

Usually, the sum of the mesiodistal measurements of mandibular molars is equal to or greater than the combined mesiodistal measurements of all the teeth anterior to the first molar and up to the median line.

The crowns of these molars are wider mesiodistally than buccolingually. The opposite is true of maxillary molars.

Mandibular First Molar

Figs. 12.1 to 12.17 illustrate the mandibular first molar from all aspects. Normally, the mandibular first molar is the largest tooth in the mandibular arch. It has five well-developed cusps: two buccal, two lingual, and one distal (see Fig. 12.1). It has two well-developed roots, one mesial and one distal, which are very broad buccolingually. These roots are widely separated at the apices.

The dimension of the crown mesiodistally is greater by about 1 mm than the dimension buccolingually (Table 12.1). Although the crown is relatively short cervico-occlusally, it has mesiodistal and buccolingual measurements that provide a broad occlusal form.

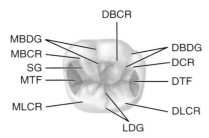

• **Fig. 12.1** Mandibular right first molar, occlusal aspect. *DBCR,* Distobuccal cusp ridge; *DBDG,* distobuccal developmental groove; *DCR,* distal cusp ridge; *DLCR,* distolingual cusp ridge; *DTF,* distal triangular fossa *(shaded area); LDG,* lingual developmental groove; *MLCR,* mesiolingual cusp ridge; *MTF,* mesial triangular fossa *(shaded area); MBCR,* mesiobuccal cusp ridge; *MBDG,* mesiobuccal developmental groove; *SG,* a supplemental groove.

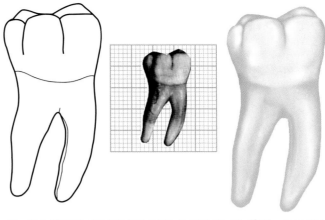

• **Fig. 12.4** Mandibular right first molar, buccal aspect. (Grid = 1 sq mm.)

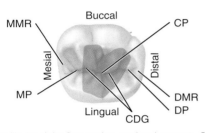

• **Fig. 12.2** Mandibular right first molar, occlusal aspect. *Shaded area* is the central fossa. *CDG,* central developmental groove; *CP,* central pit; *DMR,* distal marginal ridge; *DP,* distal pit; *MMR,* mesial marginal ridge; *MP,* mesial pit.

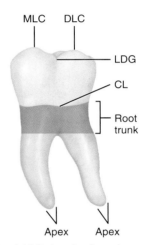

• **Fig. 12.5** Mandibular right first molar, lingual aspect. *CL,* cervical line; *DLC,* distolingual cusp; *LDG,* lingual developmental groove; *MLC,* mesiolingual cusp.

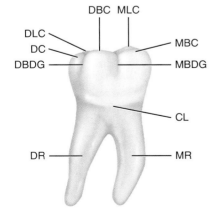

• **Fig. 12.3** Mandibular right first molar, buccal aspect. *CL,* cervical line; *DBC,* distobuccal cusp; *DBDG,* distobuccal developmental groove; *DC,* distal cusp; *DLC,* distolingual cusp; *DR,* distal root; *MBC,* mesiobuccal cusp; *MBDG,* mesiobuccal developmental groove; *MLC,* mesiolingual cusp; *MR,* mesial root.

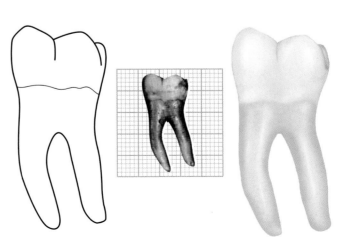

• **Fig. 12.6** Mandibular right first molar, lingual aspect. (Grid = 1 sq mm.)

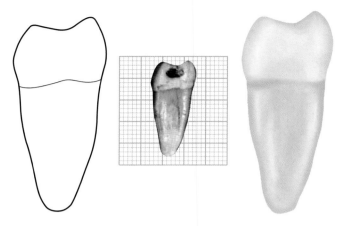

• **Fig. 12.7** Mandibular right first molar, mesial aspect. (Grid = 1 sq mm.)

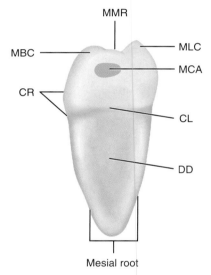

• **Fig. 12.8** Mandibular right first molar, mesial aspect. *CL,* cervical line; *CR,* cervical ridge; *DD,* developmental depression; *MBC,* mesiobuccal cusp; *MCA,* mesial contact area; *MLC,* mesiolingual cusp; *MMR,* mesial marginal ridge.

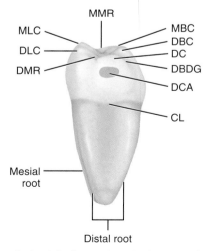

• **Fig. 12.9** Mandibular right first molar, distal aspect. *CL,* cervical line; *DBC,* distobuccal cusp; *DBDG,* distobuccal developmental groove; *DC,* distal cusp; *DCA,* distal contact area; *DLC,* distolingual cusp; *DMR,* distal marginal ridge; *MBC,* mesiobuccal cusp; *MLC,* mesiolingual cusp; *MMR,* mesial marginal ridge.

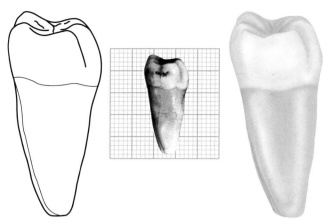

• **Fig. 12.10** Mandibular right first molar, distal aspect. (Grid = 1 sq mm.)

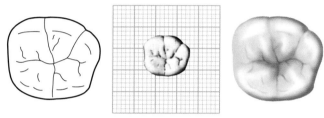

• **Fig. 12.11** Mandibular right first molar, occlusal aspect. (Grid = 1 sq mm.)

The mesial root is broad and curved distally, with mesial and distal fluting that provides the anchorage of two roots (see Fig. 13.22). The distal root is rounder, broad at the cervical portion, and pointed in a distal direction. The formation of these roots and their positions in the mandible serve to brace the crown of the tooth efficiently against the lines of force that might be brought to bear against it.

Detailed Description of the Mandibular First Molar From All Aspects

Buccal Aspect

From the buccal aspect, the crown of the mandibular first molar is roughly trapezoidal, with cervical and occlusal outlines representing the uneven sides of the trapezoid. The occlusal side is the longer (see Figs. 12.3, 12.4, and 12.12 to 12.14).

If this tooth is posed vertically, all five of its cusps are in view. The two buccal cusps and the buccal portion of the distal cusp are in the foreground, with the tips of the lingual cusps in the background. The lingual cusps may be seen because they are higher than the others.

Two developmental grooves appear on the crown portion. These grooves are called the **mesiobuccal developmental groove** and the **distobuccal developmental groove.** The first-named groove acts as a line of demarcation between the mesiobuccal lobe and the distobuccal lobe. The latter groove separates the distobuccal lobe from the distal lobe (see Figs. 12.2 and 12.3).

The mesiobuccal, distobuccal, and distal cusps are relatively flat. These cusp ridges show less curvature than those of any of the teeth described so far. The distal cusp, which is small, is more pointed than either of the buccal cusps. Flattened buccal cusps are typical of all mandibular molars. In most first molar specimens,

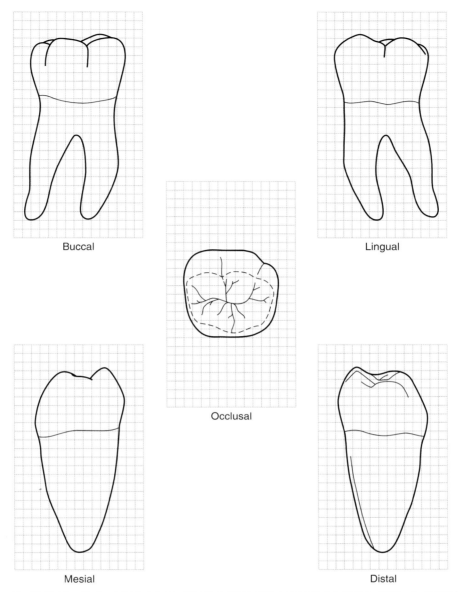

Buccal

Lingual

Occlusal

Mesial

Distal

• **Fig. 12.12** Mandibular right first molar. Graph outlines of five aspects are shown. (Grid = 1 sq mm.)

the buccal cusps are worn considerably, with the buccal cusp ridges almost at the same level. Before they are worn, the buccal cusps and the distal cusp have curvatures that are characteristic of each one (see Figs. 12.4 and 12.14, *4*).

The mesiobuccal cusp is usually the widest mesiodistally of the three cusps. This cusp has some curvature but is relatively flat. The distobuccal cusp is almost as wide, with a cusp ridge of somewhat greater curvature. The two buccal cusps make up the major portion of the buccal surface of the crown. The distal cusp provides a very small part of the buccal surface, because the major portion of the cusp makes up the distal portion of the crown, providing the distal contact area on the center of the distal surface of the distal cusp. The distal cusp ridge is very round occlusally and is sharper than either of the two buccal cusps.

These three cusps have the mesiobuccal and distobuccal grooves as lines of demarcation. The mesiobuccal groove is the shorter of the two, having its terminus centrally located cervico-occlusally. This groove is situated a little mesial to the root bifurcation buccally. The distobuccal groove has its terminus near the distobuccal

line angle at the cervical third of the crown. It travels occlusally and somewhat mesially, parallel with the axis of the distal root.

The cervical line of the mandibular first molar is commonly regular in outline, dipping apically toward the root bifurcation.

The mesial outline of the crown is somewhat concave at the cervical third up to its junction with the convex outline of the broad contact area. The distal outline of the crown is straight above the cervical line to its junction with the convex outline of the distal contact area, which is also the outline of the distal portion of the distal cusp.

The calibration of this tooth at the cervical line is 1.5 to 2 mm less mesiodistally than the mesiodistal measurement at the contact areas, which of course represents the greatest mesiodistal measurement of the crown.

The surface of the buccal portion of the crown is smoothly convex at the cusp portions with developmental grooves between the cusps. Approximately at the level of the ends of the developmental grooves, in the middle third, a developmental depression is noticeable. It runs in a mesiodistal direction just above the cervical

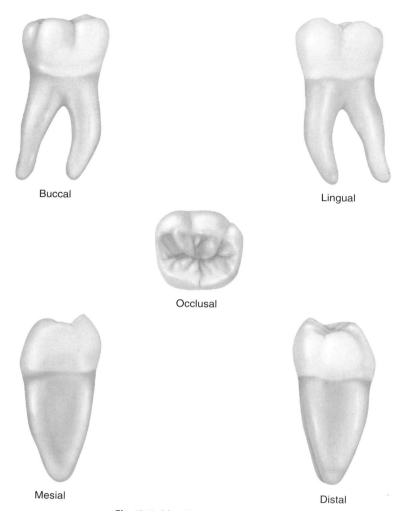

Buccal

Lingual

Occlusal

Mesial

Distal

• **Fig. 12.13** Mandibular right first molar.

ridge of the buccal surface (see Fig. 12.14, *6* and *8*). This cervical ridge may show a smooth depression in it that progresses cervically, joining with the developmental concavity just below the cervical line, which is congruent with the root bifurcation buccally.

The roots of this tooth are, in most instances, well formed and constant in development.

When the tooth is posed so that the mesiobuccal groove is directly in the line of vision, part of the distal surface of the root trunk may be seen, and in addition, part of the distal area of the mesial root is visible because the lingual portion of the root is turned distally. These areas may be seen in addition to the buccal areas of the roots and root trunk.

The mesial root is curved mesially from a point shortly below the cervical line to the middle third portion. From this point, it curves distally to the tapered apex, which is located directly below the mesiobuccal cusp. The crest of curvature of the root mesially is mesial to the crown cervix. The distal outline of the mesial root is concave from the bifurcation of the root trunk to the apex.

The distal root is less curved than the mesial root, and its axis is in a distal direction from the cervix to the apex. The root may show some curvature at its apical third in either a mesial or a distal direction (see Fig. 12.14, *1* and *8*). The apex is usually more pointed than that of the mesial root and is located below or distal to the distal contact area of the crown. Considerable variation is evident in the comparative lengths of mesial and distal roots (see Fig. 12.14).

Both roots are wider mesiodistally at the buccal areas than they are lingually. Developmental depressions are present on the mesial and distal sides of both roots, which lessens the mesiodistal measurement at those points. They are somewhat thicker at the lingual borders. This arrangement provides a secure anchorage for the mandibular first molar, preventing rotation. This I-beam principle increases the anchorage of each root (see Fig. 13.22).

The point of bifurcation of the two roots is located approximately 3 mm below the cervical line. A deep developmental depression is evident buccally on the root trunk, which starts at the bifurcation and progresses cervically, becoming shallower until it terminates at or immediately above the cervical line. This depression is smooth with no developmental groove or fold.

Lingual Aspect

From the lingual aspect, three cusps may be seen: two lingual cusps and the lingual portion of the distal cusp (see Figs. 12.5, 12.6, 12.12, and 12.13). The two lingual cusps are pointed, and the cusp ridges are high enough to hide the two buccal cusps from view. The mesiolingual cusp is the widest mesiodistally, with its cusp tip somewhat higher than the distolingual cusp. The distolingual cusp is almost as wide mesiodistally as the mesiolingual cusp. The mesiolingual and distolingual cusp ridges are inclined at angles that are similar on both lingual cusps. These cusp ridges form obtuse angles at the cusp tips of approximately 100 degrees.

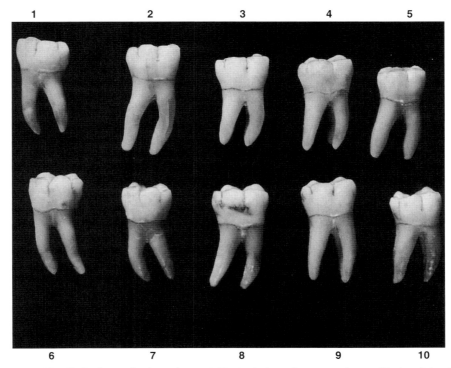

• **Fig. 12.14** Mandibular first molar, buccal aspect. Ten typical specimens are shown. (To view Animations 3 and 4 for tooth #30, please go to Expert Consult.)

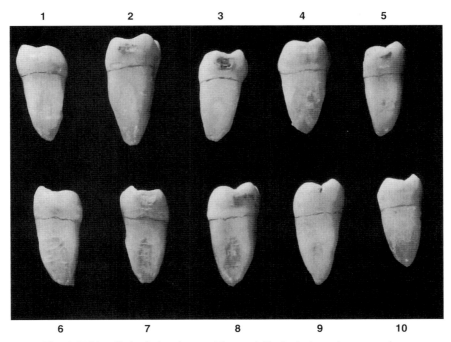

• **Fig. 12.15** Mandibular first molar, mesial aspect. Ten typical specimens are shown.

The **lingual developmental groove** serves as a line of demarcation between the lingual cusps, extending downward on the lingual surface of the crown for a short distance only. Some mandibular first molars show no groove on the lingual surface but show a depression lingual to the cusp ridges. The angle formed by the distolingual cusp ridge of the mesiolingual cusp and the mesiolingual cusp ridge of the distolingual cusp is more obtuse than the angulation of the cusp ridges at the tips of the lingual cusps.

The distal cusp is at a lower level than the mesiolingual cusp.

The mesial outline of the crown from this aspect is convex from the cervical line to the marginal ridge. The crest of contour mesially, which represents the contact area, is somewhat higher than the crest of contour distally.

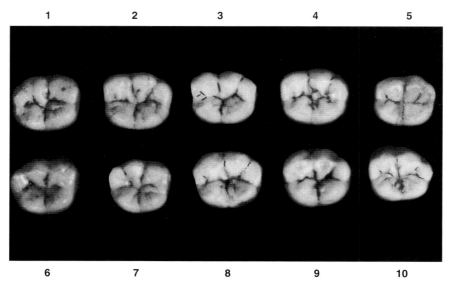

• **Fig. 12.16** Mandibular first molar, occlusal aspect. Ten typical specimens are shown.

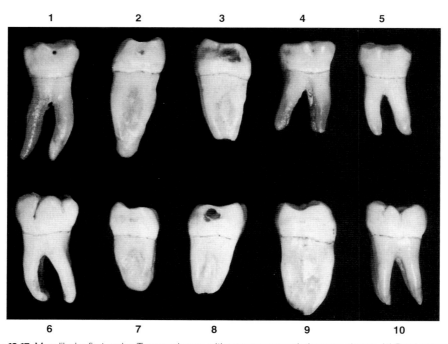

• **Fig. 12.17** Mandibular first molar. Ten specimens with uncommon variations are shown. (1) Root extremely long, crown small. (2) Mesial root longer than average with rounded apex. (3) Crown very wide buccolingually; roots short. (4) Roots short. (5) Crown has no buccal developmental grooves. (6) Crown and roots poorly formed. (7) Roots dwarfed. (8) Roots short; crown wide buccolingually. (9) Crown and root oversized buccolingually. (10) Extra tubercle or cusp attached to mesiolingual lobe.

The distal outline of the crown is straight immediately above the cervical line to a point immediately below the distal contact area; this area is represented by a convex curvature that also outlines the distal surface of the distal cusp. The junction of the distolingual cusp ridge of the distolingual cusp with the distal marginal ridge is abrupt; it gives the impression of a groove at this site from the lingual aspect. Sometimes, a shallow developmental groove occurs at this point (see Fig. 12.10). Part of the mesial and distal surfaces of the crown and root trunk may be seen from this aspect because the mesial and distal sides converge lingually.

The cervical line lingually is irregular and tends to point sharply toward the root bifurcation and immediately above it.

The surface of the crown lingually is smooth and spheroidal on each of the lingual lobes. The surface is concave at the side of the lingual groove above the center of the crown lingually. Below this point, the surface of the crown becomes almost flat as it approaches the cervical line.

The roots of the mandibular first molar appear somewhat different from the lingual aspect. They measure about 1 mm longer lingually than buccally, but the length seems more extreme (see

TABLE 12.1   Mandibular First Molar

First evidence of calcification	At birth
Enamel completed	2½–3 years
Eruption	6–7 years
Root completed	9–10 years

	MEASUREMENT TABLE							
	Cervico-Occlusal Length of Crown	Length of Root	Mesiodistal Diameter of Crown	Mesiodistal Diameter of Crown at Cervix	Labio- or Buccolingual Diameter of Crown	Labio- or Buccolingual Diameter of Crown at Cervix	Curvature of Cervical Line—Mesial	Curvature of Cervical Line—Distal
Dimensions[a] suggested for carving technique	7.5	14.0	11.0	9.0	10.5	9.0	1.0	0.0

[a]In millimeters.

Figs. 12.6 and 12.7). This impression is derived from the fact that the cusp ridges and cervical line are at a higher level (about 1 mm). This arrangement adds a millimeter to the distance from root bifurcation to the cervical line. In addition, the mesiodistal measurement of the root trunk is less toward the lingual surface than toward the buccal surface. Consequently, this slenderness lingually, in addition to the added length, makes the roots appear longer than they are from the lingual aspect (see Fig. 12.9).

As mentioned, the root bifurcation lingually starts at a point approximately 4 mm below the cervical line. This developmental depression is quite deep at this point, although it is smooth throughout and progresses cervically, becoming shallower until it fades out entirely immediately below the cervical line. The depression is rarely reflected in the cervical line or the enamel of the lingual surface of the crown, as is found in many cases on the buccal surface of this tooth.

This bifurcation groove of the root trunk is located almost in line with the lingual developmental groove of the crown.

Mesial Aspect

When the mandibular first molar is viewed from the mesial aspect, with the specimen held with its mesial surface at right angles to the line of vision, two cusps and one root only are to be seen: the mesiobuccal and mesiolingual cusps and the mesial root (see Figs. 12.7, 12.8, 12.12, 12.13, and 12.15).

The buccolingual measurement of the crown is greater at the mesial portion than it is at the distal portion. The buccolingual measurement of the mesial root is also greater than the same measurement of the distal root. Therefore, because the mesial portions of the tooth are broader and the mesial cusps are higher, the distal portions of the tooth cannot be seen from this angle.

As already indicated, all the posterior mandibular teeth have crown outlines from the mesial aspect that show a characteristic relation between crown and root. The crown from the mesial or distal aspect is roughly rhomboidal, and the entire crown has a lingual tilt in relation to the root axis. It should be remembered that the crowns of maxillary posterior teeth have the center of the occlusal surfaces between the cusps in line with the root axes (see Fig. 4.16, *E* and *F*).

It is interesting to note the difference between the *outline form of the mandibular first molar and the mandibular second premolar from the mesial aspect* (see Chapter 10). The first molar compares as follows:
1. The crown is a fraction of a millimeter to 1 mm shorter in the first molar.
2. The root is usually that much shorter as well.
3. The buccolingual measurement of crown and root of the molar is greater by 2 mm or more.
4. The lingual cusp is longer than the buccal cusp. (The opposite is true of the second premolar.)

Regardless of these differences, *the two teeth have the same functional form except for the added reinforcement given to the molar lingually.* Because of the added root width buccolingually, the buccal cusps of the first molar do not approach the center axis of the root as does the second premolar, and the lingual cusp tips are within the lingual outline of the roots instead of being on a line with them.

From the mesial aspect, the buccal outline of the crown of the mandibular first molar is convex immediately above the cervical line. Before occlusal wear has shortened the buccal cusps, this curvature is over the cervical third of the crown buccally, outlining the **buccal cervical ridge** (see Fig. 12.8). This ridge is more prominent on some first molars than on others (see Fig. 12.15). Just as on mandibular premolars, this ridge curvature does not exceed similar contours on other teeth as a rule when the mandibular first molar is posed in the position it assumes in the mandibular arch (see Fig. 12.7 and Fig. 12.15, *1* and *2*).

Above the buccal cervical ridge, the outline of the buccal contour may be slightly concave on some specimens (see Fig. 12.15, *1* and *2*), or the outline may just be less convex or even rather flat as it continues occlusally outlining the contour of the mesiobuccal cusp. The mesiobuccal cusp is located directly above the buccal third of the mesial root.

The lingual outline of the crown is straight in a lingual direction, starting at the cervical line and joining the lingual curvature at the middle third, the lingual curvature being pronounced between this point and the tip of the mesiolingual cusp. The crest of the lingual contour is located at the center of the middle third of the crown. The tip of the mesiolingual cusp is in a position directly above the lingual third of the mesial root.

The mesial marginal ridge is confluent with the mesial ridges of the mesiobuccal and mesiolingual cusps. The marginal ridge is placed about 1 mm below the level of the cusp tips.

The cervical line mesially is rather irregular and tends to curve occlusally about 1 mm toward the center of the mesial surface of the tooth (see Fig. 12.15, *1, 4, 9,* and *10*). The cervical line may assume a relatively straight line buccolingually (see Fig. 12.15, *3, 6,* and *8*).

In all instances, the cervical line is at a higher level lingually than buccally, usually about 1 mm higher. The difference in level may be greater. This relation depends on the assumption that the tooth is posed vertically. When the first molar is in its normal position in the lower jaw, leaning to the lingual, the cervical line is nearly level buccolingually.

The surface of the crown is convex and smooth over the mesial contours of the mesiolingual and mesiobuccal lobes. A flattened or slightly concave area exists at the cervical line immediately above the center of the mesial root. This area is right below the contact area and joins the concavity of the central portion of the root at the cervix. The contact area is almost centered buccolingually in the mesial surface of the crown, and it is placed below the crest of the marginal ridge about one-third the distance from the marginal ridge to the cervical line. (See stained contact area on specimen in Fig. 12.7. Before contact wear has occurred, the contact area is not as broad. Refer also to Fig. 12.4.)

The buccal outline of the mesial root drops straight down from the cervical line buccally to a point near the junction of the cervical and middle thirds of the root. A gentle curve starts lingually from this point to the apex, which is located directly below the mesiobuccal cusp.

The lingual outline of the mesial root is slanted in a buccal direction, although the outline is nearly straight from the cervical line lingually to the point of junction of middle and apical thirds of the root. From this point, the curvature is sharply buccal to the bluntly tapered apex. On those specimens that show a short bifurcation at the mesial root end, the curvature at the apical third lingually is slight (see Fig. 12.15, *2* and *10*).

The mesial surface of the mesial root is convex at the buccal and lingual borders, with a broad concavity between these convexities the full length of the root from the cervical line to the apex. If a specimen tooth is held in front of a strong light so that the distal side of the mesial root can be seen from the apical aspect, it is noted that the same contours exist on the root distally as are found mesially, and the root is very thin where the concavities are superimposed. The root form appears to be two narrow roots fused together with thin, hard tissue between.

The mesial surface of the distal root is smooth, with no deep developmental depressions.

Distal Aspect

Because the gross outline of the distal aspect of the crown and root of the mandibular first molar is similar to that from the mesial aspect, the description of outline form will not be repeated. When this aspect is considered from the standpoint of a three-dimensional figure, however, more of the tooth is seen from the distal aspect, because the crown is shorter distally than mesially and the buccal and lingual surfaces of the crown converge distally (see Figs. 12.10, 12.12, and 12.13). The buccal surface shows more convergence than the lingual surface. The distal root is narrower buccolingually than the mesial root.

If a specimen of the first molar is held with the distal surface of the crown at right angles to the line of vision, a great part of the occlusal surface may be seen and some part of each of the five cusps also, which compares favorably with the mandibular second premolar. This is caused in part by the placement of the crowns on the roots with a distal inclination to the long axes. The slight variation in crown length distally does not provide this view of the occlusal surface (see Figs. 12.9 and 12.10).

From the distal aspect, the distal cusp is in the foreground on the crown portion. The distal cusp is placed a little buccal to the center buccolingually, with the distal contact area appearing on its distal contour.

The distal contact area is placed just below the distal cusp ridge of the distal cusp and at a slightly higher level above the cervical line than was found mesially compared with the location of the mesial contact area.

The distal marginal ridge is short and is made up of the distal cusp ridge of the distal cusp and the distolingual cusp ridge of the distolingual cusp. These cusp ridges dip sharply in a cervical direction, meeting at an obtuse angle. Often, a developmental groove or depression is found crossing the marginal ridge at this point. The point of this angle is above the lingual third of the distal root instead of being centered over the root as is true of the center of the mesial marginal ridge.

The distal contact area is centered over the distal root; this arrangement places it buccal to the center point of the distal marginal ridge.

The surface of the distal portion of the crown is convex on the distal cusp and the distolingual cusp. Contact wear may produce a flattened area at the point of contact on the distal surface of the distal cusp. Just above the cervical line, the enamel surface is flat where it joins the flattened surface of the root trunk distally.

The cervical line distally usually extends straight across buccolingually. It may be irregular, dipping rootwise just below the distal contact area (see Fig. 12.10).

The end of the distobuccal developmental groove is located on the distal surface and forms a concavity at the cervical portion of the distobuccal line angle of the crown. The distal portion of the crown extends out over the root trunk distally at quite an angle (see Fig. 12.4). The smooth, flat surface below the contact area remains fairly constant to the apical third of the distal root. Sometimes a developmental depression is found here. The apical third portion of the root is more rounded as it tapers to a sharper apex than is found on the mesial root.

The lingual border of the mesial root may be seen from the distal aspect.

Occlusal Aspect

The mandibular first molar is somewhat hexagonal from the occlusal aspect (see Fig. 12.2). The crown measurement is greater by 1 mm or more mesiodistally than buccolingually. It must be remembered that the opposite arrangement is true of the maxillary first molar.

The buccolingual measurement of the crown is greater on the mesial than on the distal side. Also, the measurement of the crown at the contact areas, which includes the two buccal cusps and the distal cusp, is greater than the mesiodistal measurement of the two lingual cusps. In other words, the crown converges lingually from the contact areas. This convergence varies in individual specimens (see Fig. 12.16, *1* and *4*).

It is interesting to note the degree of development of the individual cusps from the occlusal aspect (see Figs. 12.1, 12.2, 12.11 to 12.13, and 12.16). The mesiobuccal cusp is slightly larger than either of the two lingual cusps, which are almost equal to each other in size; the distobuccal cusp is smaller than any one of the other three mentioned, and the distal cusp is in most cases the smallest of all.

More variance is evident in the development of the distobuccal and distal lobes than in any of the others (see Fig. 12.16, *1, 7,* and *10*).

When the tooth is posed so that the line of vision is parallel with the long axis, a great part of the buccal surface may be seen, whereas only a small portion of the lingual surface may be seen lingual to the lingual cusp ridges. No part of the mesial or distal surfaces is in view below the outline of the mesial and distal marginal ridges. (Compare tooth outlines from the other aspects.)

All mandibular molars, including the first molar, are essentially quadrilateral in form. The mandibular first molar, in most instances, has a functioning distal cusp, although it is small in comparison with the other cusps. Occasionally, four-cusp first molars are found, and more often, one discovers first molars with distobuccal and distal cusps showing fusion with little or no trace of a distobuccal developmental groove between them (see Fig. 12.16, *1* and Fig. 12.17, *4* and *5*). *From a developmental viewpoint, all mandibular molars have four major cusps, whereas maxillary molars have only three major cusps* (see Fig. 11.11).

The occlusal surfaces of the mandibular first molar may be described as follows: there is a major fossa and two minor fossae. The major fossa is the central fossa (see Fig. 12.2). It is roughly circular, and it is centrally placed on the occlusal surface between buccal and lingual cusp ridges. The two minor fossae are the **mesial triangular fossa,** immediately distal to the mesial marginal ridge, and the **distal triangular fossa,** immediately mesial to the distal marginal ridge (see Fig. 12.1).

The developmental grooves on the occlusal surface are the **central developmental groove,** the *mesiobuccal developmental groove,* the *distobuccal developmental groove,* and the *lingual developmental groove.* Supplemental grooves, accidental short grooves, and developmental pits are also found. Most of the supplemental grooves are tributary to the developmental grooves within the bounds of cusp ridges.

The central fossa of the occlusal surface is a concave area bounded by the distal slope of the mesiobuccal cusp, both mesial and distal slopes of the distobuccal cusp, the mesial slope of the distal cusp, the distal slope of the mesiolingual cusp, and the mesial slope of the distolingual cusp (see Fig. 12.2).

All of the developmental grooves converge in the center of the central fossa at the **central pit.**

The *mesial triangular fossa* of the occlusal surface is a smaller concave area than the central fossa, and the mesial slope of the mesiobuccal cusp, the mesial marginal ridge, and the mesial slope of the mesiolingual cusp bound it. The mesial portion of the central developmental groove terminates in this fossa. Usually a buccal and a lingual supplemental groove join it at a **mesial pit** within the boundary of the mesial marginal ridge. Sometimes a supplemental groove crosses the mesial marginal ridge lingual to the contact area (see Fig. 12.16, *2, 8, 9,* and *10*).

The *distal triangular fossa* is in most instances less distinct than the mesial fossa. The distal slope of the distal cusp, the distal marginal ridge, and the distal slope of the distolingual cusp bound it.

The central groove has its other terminal in this fossa. Buccal and lingual supplemental grooves are less common here. An extension of the central groove quite often crosses the distal marginal ridge, however, lingual to the distal contact area.

Starting at the central pit in the central fossa, the central developmental groove travels an irregular course mesially, terminating in the mesial triangular fossa. A short distance mesially from the central pit, it joins the mesiobuccal developmental groove. The latter groove courses in a mesiobuccal direction at the bottom of a sulcate groove separating the mesiobuccal and distobuccal cusps. At the junction of the cusp ridges of those cusps, the mesiobuccal groove of the occlusal surface is confluent with the mesiobuccal groove of the buccal surface of the crown. The lingual developmental groove of the occlusal surface is an irregular groove coursing in a lingual direction at the bottom of the lingual sulcate groove to the junction of lingual cusp ridges, where it is confluent with the lingual extension of the same groove. Again starting at the central pit, the central groove may be followed in a distobuccal direction to a point where it is joined by the distobuccal developmental groove of the occlusal surface. From this point, the central groove courses in a distolingual direction, terminating in the distal triangular fossa. The distobuccal groove passes from its junction with the central groove in a distobuccal course, joining its buccal extension on the buccal surface of the crown at the junction of the cusp ridges of the distobuccal and distal cusps.

The central developmental groove seems to be centrally located in relation to the buccolingual crown dimension. This arrangement makes the triangular ridges of lingual cusps longer than the triangular ridges of buccal cusps.

Note the relative position and relative size of the distal cusp from the occlusal aspect. The distal portion of it joins the distal contact area of the crown.

Mandibular Second Molar

Figs. 12.18 to 12.26 illustrate the mandibular second molar from all aspects. The mandibular second molar supplements the first molar in function. Its anatomy differs in some details.

Normally, the second molar is smaller than the first molar by a fraction of a millimeter in all dimensions (Table 12.2). It does not, however, run true to form. It is not uncommon to find mandibular second molar crowns somewhat larger than first molar crowns, and although the roots are not as well formed, they may be longer.

The crown has four well-developed cusps, two buccal and two lingual, of nearly equal development. Neither a distal nor a fifth cusp is evident, but the distobuccal cusp is larger than that found on the first molar.

The tooth has two well-developed roots, one mesial and one distal. These roots are broad buccolingually, but they are not as broad as those of the first molar, nor are they as widely separated.

Detailed Description of the Mandibular Second Molar From All Aspects

In describing this tooth, direct comparisons will be made with the first mandibular molar. Uncommon variations are shown in Figure 12.26.

Buccal Aspect

From the buccal aspect the crown is somewhat shorter cervico-occlusally and narrower mesiodistally than is the first molar (see Fig. 12.18). The crown and root show a tendency toward

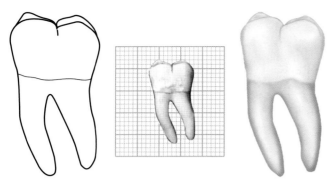

• **Fig. 12.18** Mandibular left second molar, buccal aspect. (Grid = 1 sq mm.)

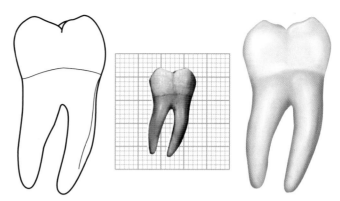

• **Fig. 12.19** Mandibular left second molar, lingual aspect. (Grid = 1 sq mm.)

greater overall length but are not always longer (see Fig. 12.23, *4, 7,* and *9*). (To view Animations 3 and 4, please go to Expert Consult.)

Only one developmental groove lies buccally—the buccal developmental groove. This groove acts as a line of demarcation between the mesiobuccal and the distobuccal cusps, which are about equal in their mesiodistal measurements.

The cervical line buccally in many instances points sharply toward the root bifurcation (see Fig. 12.23, *1, 2, 3, 5,* and *9*).

The roots may be shorter than those of the first molar, but they vary considerably in this and in their development generally. The roots are usually closer together, and their axes are nearly parallel. They may spread as much as those of the first molar (see Fig. 12.23, *5*), or they may be fused for all or part of their length (see Fig. 12.23, *8* and *9*).

The roots are inclined distally in relation to the occlusal plane of the crown, their axes forming more of an acute angle with the occlusal plane than is found on the first molar. When one compares all of the mandibular molars, it may seem that the first molar shows one angulation of roots to occlusal plane, the second molar shows a more acute angle, and the third molar shows an angle that is more acute still (see Fig. 16.20).

Lingual Aspect

Differences in detail between the mandibular second molar and the mandibular first molar, to be noted from the lingual aspect (see Fig. 12.19), are as follows:

1. The crown and root of the mandibular second molar converge lingually but to a slight degree; little of the mesial or distal surfaces may therefore be seen from this aspect.
2. The mesiodistal calibration at the cervix lingually is always greater accordingly than that of the first molar.
3. The curvatures mesially and distally on the crown that describe the contact areas are more noticeable from the lingual aspect. They prove to be at a slightly lower level, especially in the distal area, than those of the first molar.

Mesial Aspect

Except for the differences in measurement from the mesial aspect, the second molar differs little from the first molar (see Figs. 12.20 and 12.24).

The cervical ridge buccally on the crown portion is in most instances less pronounced, and the occlusal surface may be more constricted buccolingually (see Fig. 12.24, *2, 8,* and *10*).

The cervical line shows less curvature, being straight and regular in outline buccolingually.

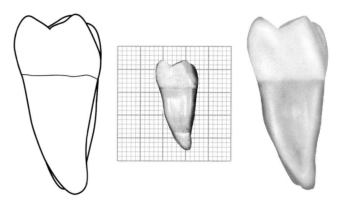

• **Fig. 12.20** Mandibular left second molar, mesial aspect. (Grid = 1 sq mm.)

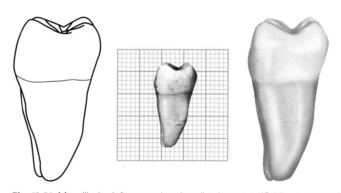

• **Fig. 12.21** Mandibular left second molar, distal aspect. (Grid = 1 sq mm.)

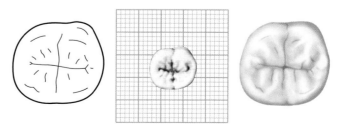

• **Fig. 12.22** Mandibular left second molar, occlusal aspect. (Grid = 1 sq mm.)

It is possible for any root of a tooth to have multiple apical foramina. If these openings are large enough, the space that leads to the main root canal is called a **supplementary** or **lateral canal** (Fig. 13.5). If the root canal breaks up into multiple tiny canals, it is referred to as a *delta system*[2] because of its complexity (Fig. 13.6).

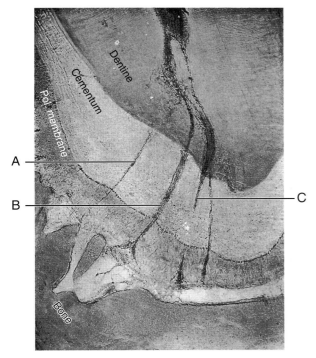

• **Fig. 13.5** A section through the apex of a root showing multiple canals (*A* through *C*). Three canals are present within the dentin, but one canal divides at the cementum-dentin junction *(C)*, which makes a total of four small canals that exit on the cemental surface of the tooth (Talbot).

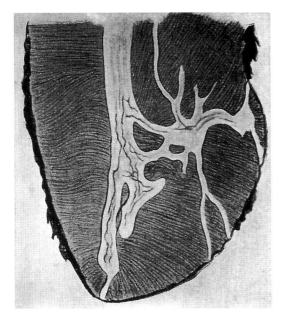

• **Fig. 13.6** Apical end of root showing one main canal and an adjacent delta system. (From Riethmuller RH: The filling of root canals with Prinz' paraffin compound, *Dent Cosmos* 56:490, 1914.)

Demarcation of Pulp Cavity and Canal

The cementoenamel junction (CEJ) is not quite at the level at which the root canal becomes the pulp chamber (see Fig. 13.1). This demarcation is mainly macroscopically based but may be visualized by exploring the CEJ (see Fig. 2.15) and noting the difference in density between the enamel and dentin at the mesial and distal tooth surfaces on radiographs. Enamel covers the external surface of the dentin, which makes up part of the pulp chamber, whereas cementum covers the entire external dentinal surface of the root canal space. The demarcation is simpler in multirooted teeth because the pulp cavity within the root is the root canal and the remaining pulp cavity is the pulp chamber. Microscopically, the pulp within the chamber appears to be more cellular than the pulp found within the pulp of the root canal. The odontoblasts are cuboidal in the coronal pulp chamber but gradually flatten out as the apex is approached. The transition from the pulp chamber to the root canal is not sharply demarcated microscopically and this demarcation is not sharply delineated macroscopically.

Pulp Horns

Projections or prolongations in the roof of the pulp chamber correspond to the various major cusps or lobes of the crown. The pulpal tissues that occupy these prolongations are called **pulp horns** (Fig. 13.7). The prominence of the cusps or lobes corresponds to the development of the pulp horns. If the cusps or labial lobes are prominent (as in young individuals), one should expect to find equally prominent pulp horns underlying these structures (Fig. 13.8B, *6*). These projections become less prominent with time as a result of the formation of secondary dentin (see Fig. 13.8B, *1*).

Clinical Applications

One of the primary functions of the dentist is to prevent, intercept, and treat diseases or disorders affecting the dentition. It is also essential that the clinician be aware of the location and size of the pulp cavities during operative procedures in order to prevent unnecessary encroachment on the pulp. It is also incumbent on the clinician to know the location of the mandibular canal and nerve.

Endodontic procedures also require a thorough knowledge of the pulp cavity. Perforation during access preparation, failure to locate all the canals, or perforation of the root surface may ultimately result in loss of the tooth. Therefore the clinician performing endodontics must know the size and location of the pulp chamber and the expected number of roots and canals. Likewise, the clinician must be aware of variations in racial groups or in individuals within the same race. The presence of extra roots and C-shaped canals are examples found in some studies.[3]

Radiographic detection of all accessory roots or canals may not be possible, although there is some evidence that additional canals are present based on the shape of the crown. Even so, the clinician must recognize some of the internal signs of additional canals during the endodontic procedure. With a thorough knowledge of the pulp cavities in the permanent dentition, prevention, interception, and treatment of dentition-related disease processes will be accomplished with a greater degree of success.

Pulp Cavities of the Maxillary Teeth

Maxillary Central Incisor

Labiolingual Section (see Fig. 13.8A)

The pulp cavity follows the general outline of the crown and root. The pulp chamber is very narrow in the incisal region. If a great amount

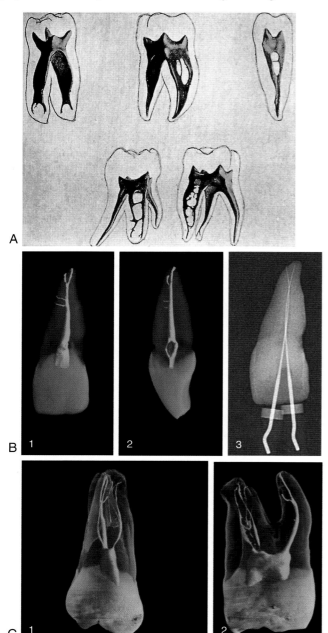

A

B 1 2 3

C 1 2

• **Fig. 13.7** (A) Molar and bicuspid pulp cavities. Note the prominence of the pulp horns and the complexities of the pulp chambers and root canal systems. (B) Microcomputed tomographic scans of dental anatomy (36-μm resolution). *1*, Clinical view of tooth #9 shows two accessory canals and an apical bifurcation. *2*, Mesiodistal view of the tooth shown in 1. *3*, Working-length radiograph with files placed in both apical canal aspects. (C) Microcomputed tomographic scans of more complicated dental anatomy (36-μm resolution). *1*, Clinical view of tooth #3 shows a fine mesiobuccal and distobuccal canal system with additional anatomy in all three roots. *2*, Mesiodistal view of the tooth shown in 1. (A, From Riethmuller RH: The filling of root canals with Prinz' paraffin compound, *Dent Cosmos* 56:490, 1914. B and C, From Cohen S, Hargreaves KM: *Pathways of the pulp*, ed 9, St Louis, 2006, Mosby.)

of secondary or irritation-induced dentin has been produced, this portion of the pulp chamber may be partially or completely obliterated (see Fig. 13.8A, *3*). In the cervical region of the tooth, the pulp chamber increases to its largest labiolingual dimension.

Below the cervical area, the root canal tapers, gradually ending in a constriction at the apex of the tooth (apical constriction). The apical foramen is usually located near the very tip of the root but may be located slightly to the labial (see Fig. 13.8A, *3* to *5*) or lingual aspect of the root (see Fig. 13.8A, *1* and *6*). Because of this generalized phenomenon, it has been suggested that the root canal filling should appear on radiographs to extend no closer than 1 mm from the radiographic apex of the tooth. However, with the use of an electronic apical locator, the clinician can be surer of reaching the apex more closely without overfilling.

Mesiodistal Section (see Fig. 13.8B)

The pulp chamber is wider in the mesiodistal than in the labiolingual dimension. The pulp cavity conforms to the general shape of the outer surface of the tooth. If prominent mamelons (see Fig. 1.10B) are or have been present, it is not unusual to find definite prolongations or pulp horns in the incisal region of the tooth (see Fig. 13.8B, *5* and *6*). The pulp cavity then tapers rather evenly along its entire length until it reaches the apical constriction. The position of the apical foramen is usually slightly off center from the tip of the root, but some foramina deviate drastically from the apex of the root (see Fig. 13.8B, *6*).

Cervical and Midroot Cross Sections (see Fig. 13.8C and D)

The pulp cavity is widest at about the cervical level, and the pulp chamber is generally centered within the dentin of the root (Fig. 13.8C, *1* to *5*). In young individuals the pulp chamber is roughly triangular in outline, with the base of the triangle at the labial aspect of the root (see Fig. 13.8C, *5*). As the amount of secondary or reactive dentin increases, the pulp chamber becomes more round or crescent-shaped (see Fig. 13.8C, *3*, *4*, and *6*). The outline form of the root at the cervical level is typically triangular with rounded corners (see Fig. 13.8C, *5* and *6*), but some are more rectangular or angular with rounded corners (see Fig. 13.8C, *1* to *4*). The root and pulp canal tend to be rounder at the midroot level (see Fig 13.8D, *1* to *6*) than at the cervical level. The anatomy at the midroot level is essentially the same as that found at the cervical level; it is just smaller in all dimensions.

Maxillary Lateral Incisor

Labiolingual Section (Fig. 13.9A)

The anatomy of the lateral incisor is similar to that of the central incisor. The pulp cavity of the lateral incisor generally follows the outline form of the crown and the root. The pulp horns are usually prominent. The pulp chamber is narrow in the incisal region and may become very wide at the cervical level of the tooth (see Fig. 13.9A, *1* to *3* and *5*). Those teeth lacking this cervical enlargement of the pulp chamber possess a root canal that tapers slightly to the apical constriction (see Fig. 13.9A, *4* and *6*). Many of the apical foramina appear to be located at the tip of the root in the labiolingual aspect (see Fig. 13.9A, *1*, *4*, and *6*), whereas some exit on the labial (see Fig. 13.9A, *2* and *3*) or lingual aspect of the root tip (see Fig. 13.9A, *5*).

Mesiodistal Section (see Fig. 13.9B)

The pulp cavity closely follows the external outline of the tooth. The pulpal projections or pulp horns appear to be blunted when viewed from the labial aspect of the tooth. The pulp chamber and root canal gradually taper toward the apex, which often

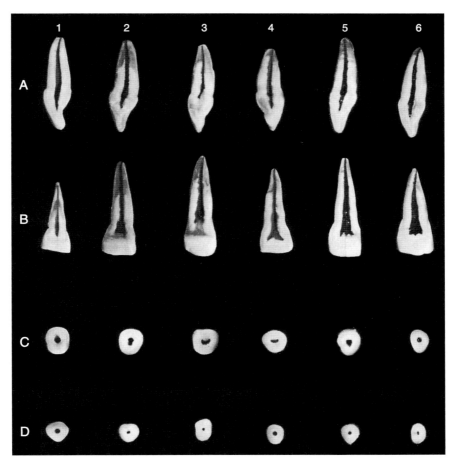

• **Fig. 13.8** Maxillary central incisor. Sections of natural specimens. (A) *1* through *6*, Labiolingual sections. This aspect does not appear in the radiographs. (B) *1* through *6*, mesiodistal sections. (C) *1* through *6*, cervical cross sections of root. (D) *1* through *6*, midroot cross sections.

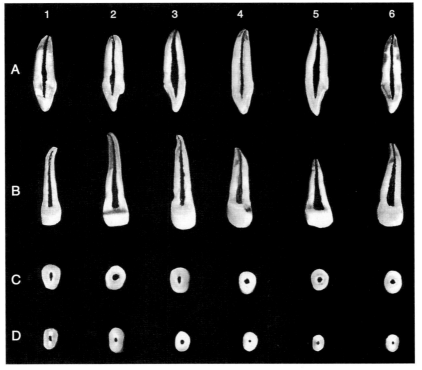

• **Fig. 13.9** Maxillary lateral incisor. Sections of natural specimens. (A) *1* through *6*, labiolingual sections. This aspect does not appear in the radiographs. (B) *1* through *6*, mesiodistal sections. (C) *1* through *6*, cervical cross sections of root. (D) *1* through *6*, midroot cross sections.

demonstrates a significant curve toward the distal in the apical region (see Fig. 13.9B, *1* to *4* and *6*).

Cervical and Midroot Cross Sections (see Fig. 13.9C and D)

The cervical cross section shows the pulp chamber to be centered within the root. The root form of this tooth shows a large variation in shape (see the discussion of the lateral incisor in Chapter 6). The outline form of this tooth may be triangular, oval, or round (see Fig. 13.9C, *1* to *6*). The pulp chamber generally follows the outline form of the root, but secondary dentin may narrow the canal significantly (see Fig. 13.9D, *4* and *6*).

Maxillary Canine

Labiolingual Section (Fig. 13.10A and D)

The maxillary canine has the largest labiolingual root dimension of any tooth in the mouth. Because the pulp cavity corresponds closely to the outline of the tooth, the pulp chamber of this tooth may also be the largest in the mouth.

The incisal aspect of the canine corresponds to the shape of the crown. If a prominent cusp is present, a long narrow projection from the pulp chamber (the pulp horn) will be present. The pulp chamber and incisal third or half of the root canal may be very wide, showing a very abrupt constriction of the root canal in the apical region, which then gently tapers toward the apex (see Fig 13.10A, *4* to *6*, and *8*; D, *16* to *18*). In other instances a root canal may taper evenly from the pulp chamber to the apex of the root (see Fig. 13.10A, *9*; D, *10*, *11*, *13*, and *14*).

Some canines have severe curves in the apical aspect of the root (see Fig. 13.10A, *3* and *7*). The apical foramen may appear to exit at the tip of the root (see Fig. 13.10A, *2* and *5* through *8*; D, *11*, *17*, and *18*) or labially to the apex of the root (see Fig. 13.10A, *1*, *3*, and *4*; D, *12* to *16*).

Mesiodistal Section (see Fig. 13.10B and E)

The pulp cavity is much narrower in the mesiodistal aspect. The dimension and degree of taper of the pulp canal of the maxillary canine are very similar to those of the central and lateral incisors;

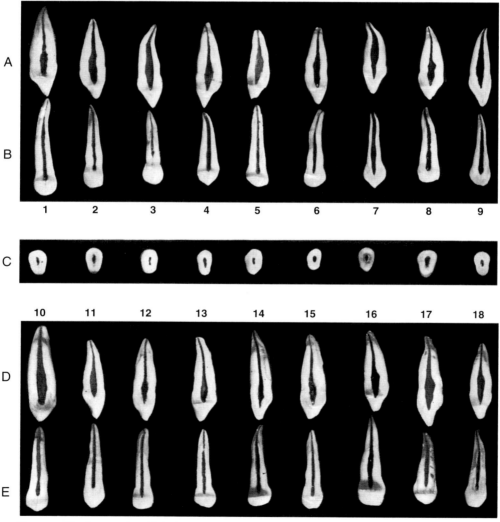

• **Fig. 13.10** Maxillary canine. (A) Labiolingual section, exposing the mesial or distal aspect of the pulp cavity. This aspect does not appear on dental radiographs. (B) Mesiodistal section, exposing the labial or lingual aspect of the pulp cavity. (C) Cervical cross section at the cementoenamel junction, exposing the pulp chamber. These are the openings to root canals that will be seen in the floor of the pulp chamber. (D) Labiolingual section, exposing the mesial or distal aspect of the pulp cavity. (E) Mesiodistal section, exposing the labial or lingual aspect of the pulp cavity.

however, the cuspid has a much longer root. The pulp cavity gently tapers from the incisal aspect to the apical foramen. A mesial or distal curve of the apical root may be present (see Fig. 13.10B, *1, 4, 6,* and *8;* E, *14, 17,* and *18*). The apical foramen may appear to exit at the tip of the root (see Fig. 13.10B, *1, 3* to *5, 7,* and *9;* E, *10, 11, 13, 14, 17,* and *18*) or slightly to its mesial or distal aspect (see Fig. 13.10B, *2, 6,* and *8;* E, *12, 15,* and *16*).

Cervical Cross Section (see Fig. 13.10C)

In a cervical cross section, the shape of the root and pulp cavity is oval (see Fig. 13.10C, *6, 7,* and *9*), triangular (see Fig. 13.10C, *8*), or elliptical (see Fig. 13.10C, *1* to *5*). The pulp chamber and canal are often centered within the crown and root (see Fig. 13.10C, *1, 3, 4,* and *9*).

Maxillary First Premolar

Buccolingual Section (Fig. 13.11A and D)

The maxillary first premolar may have two well-developed roots (see Fig. 13.11A, *1, 2,* and *9;* D, *10* and *14*), two root projections that are not fully separated (see Fig. 13.11A, *3, 5, 7,* and *8;* D, *11*

to *13* and *15* to *17*), or one broad root (see Fig. 13.11A, *4* and *6;* D, *18*). The majority of maxillary first premolars have two root canals (see Fig. 13.11A and D). A small percentage of maxillary first premolar teeth may have three roots that may be almost undetectable radiographically.

The pulp horn usually extends further incisally under the buccal cusp, because this cusp is usually better developed than the lingual cusp. The pulp horns may be blunted (see Fig. 13.11A, *1, 5,* and *6;* D, *11*) in teeth possessing cusps that demonstrate a fair amount of attrition. The pulp chamber's floor is below the cervical level of all the variations found in the maxillary first premolar. The pulp chamber of teeth having the least root separation usually shows the largest incisal-apical dimension (see Fig. 13.11A, *4;* D, *18*). Those teeth possessing a partial root separation may also have this large dimension (see Fig. 13.11A, *8;* D, *10*). Teeth having two separate canals usually demonstrate a rather small pulp chamber in the incisal-apical direction (see Fig. 13.11A, *1, 2,* and *9;* D, *11* and *14*). The shape of the pulp chamber (excluding the pulp horns) tends to be square (see Fig. 13.11A, *1* and *8;* D, *10, 12, 13, 14,* and *18*) or rectangular (see Fig. 13.11A, *2* to *7;* D, *11, 15, 16,* and *17*).

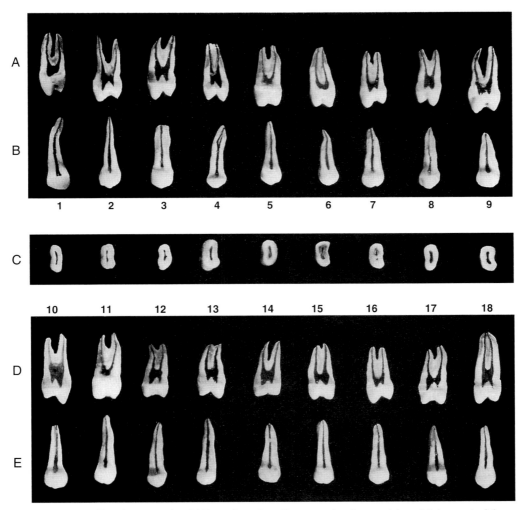

• **Fig. 13.11** Maxillary first premolar. (A) Buccolingual section, exposing the mesial or distal aspect of the pulp cavity. This aspect does not appear on the dental radiographs. (B) Mesiodistal section, exposing the buccal or lingual aspect of the pulp cavity. (C) Cervical cross section at the cementoenamel junction, exposing the pulp chamber. These are the openings to root canals that will be seen in the floor of the pulp chamber. (D) Buccolingual section, exposing the mesial or distal aspect of the pulp cavity. (E) Mesiodistal section, exposing the buccal or lingual aspect of the pulp cavity.

The root canal often appears to exit at the tip of the root (see Fig. 13.11A, *1, 4, 6, 7,* and *8;* B, *12, 13,* and *15* to *18*), slightly to the labial or lingual (see Fig. 13.11A, *2*), or a combination of the two locations (see Fig. 13.11A, *3, 5,* and *9;* B, *10, 11,* and *14*).

Mesiodistal Section (see Fig. 13.11B and E)

The pulp horns appear blunted from the mesial or distal aspect, and the pulp chamber cannot be differentiated from the root canal. The pulp cavity tapers slightly from the occlusal aspect to the apical foramen. If two canals are present, the radiopacity will increase in the apical half of the tooth because of an increased amount of dentin and bone and a decrease in the volume of the pulp cavity.

The apical foramen appears to exit at the tip of the root most of the time (see Fig. 13.11B, *1, 2, 3,* and *6* through *9;* E, *10* and *12* through *18*), but some appear to exit on the mesial or distal aspects of the root (see Fig. 13.11B, *4* and *5;* E, *11*).

Cervical Cross Section (see Fig. 13.11C)

The cross section at the cervical level shows the kidney-shaped outline form characteristic of the maxillary first premolar (see Fig. 13.11C). A mesial developmental groove is usually present, giving

this tooth its classic indentation. The pulp cavity may demonstrate a constriction adjacent to the developmental groove (see Fig. 13.11C, *2, 3, 5, 6,* and *9*), or it may follow the general outline of the root surface (see Fig. 13.11C, *1, 4, 7,* and *8*). Some roots demonstrate two separate root canals (see Fig. 13.11C, *7*), whereas a cross section of a three-rooted maxillary first premolar will show three separate canals (see Fig. 13.11C, *3*).

Maxillary Second Premolar

Buccolingual Section (Fig. 13.12A and D)

Most maxillary second premolars have only one root and one canal. Two roots are possible, although two canals within a single root may also be found.

The pulp cavity may demonstrate well-developed pulp horns (see Fig. 13.12A, *1, 2, 6, 7,* and *8;* D, *10, 11, 12, 14, 16,* and *17*); others may have blunted or nonexistent pulp horns (see Fig. 13.12A, *3, 4, 5,* and *9;* D, *13, 15,* and *18*). The pulp chamber and root canal are very broad in the buccolingual aspect of teeth with single canals. The pulp cavity does not show a well-defined demarcation between the root cavity and the pulp cavity because of the large buccolingual extent of the pulp cavity in the upper half of

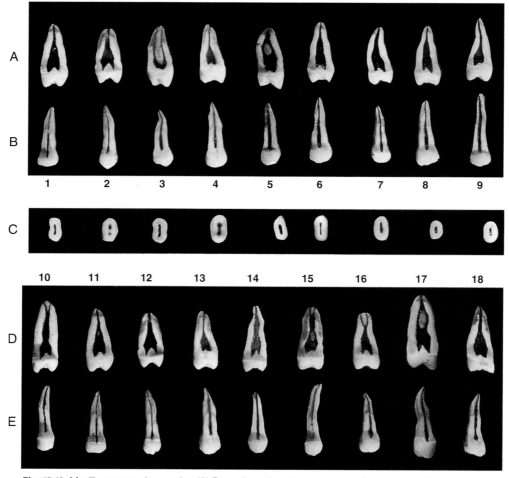

• **Fig. 13.12** Maxillary second premolar. (A) Buccolingual section, exposing the mesial or distal aspect of the pulp cavity. This aspect does not appear on the dental radiographs. (B) Mesiodistal section, exposing the buccal or lingual aspect of the pulp cavity. (C) Cervical cross section at the cementoenamel junction, exposing the pulp chamber. These are the openings to root canals that will be seen in the floor of the pulp chamber. (D) Buccolingual section, exposing the mesial or distal aspect of the pulp cavity. (E) Mesiodistal section, exposing the buccal or lingual aspect of the pulp cavity.

Mesiodistal Section (see Fig. 13.23B and E)

The mesiodistal sections of the mandibular second molar are very similar to those of the mandibular first molar. However, the roots of the mandibular first molar tend to be straighter and closer together (less furcation deviation).

The pulp horns are usually prominent (see Fig. 13.23B, *1, 2, 3, 5, 7, 8,* and *9*; E, *10, 11, 13, 15,* and *18*), but some are small or absent (see Fig. 13.23B, *4* and *6*; E, *12, 14, 16,* and *17*).

The pulp chamber is rectangular (excluding the pulp horns). The size of the chamber varies from very large (see Fig. 13.23B, *1, 3, 4, 5, 7,* and *9*; E, *13* and *16*) to very small (see Fig. 13.23B, *2* and *8*; E, *11, 14, 17,* and *18*).

The curvature of the mesial canal may be severe (see Fig. 13.23B, *3, 6, 8,* and *9*; E, *11, 14, 16,* and *17*), moderate (see Fig. 13.23B, *2, 4,* and *7*; E, *10, 13, 15,* and *18*), or essentially straight (see Fig. 13.23B, *1* and *5*; E, *12*). The canals gently taper from the pulp chamber to the apical constriction.

The apical foramen usually appears to be located at the tip of the root (see Fig. 13.23B, *2, 4* through *7,* and *8*; E, *11, 12, 13, 15, 17,* and *18*), but the foramen may appear to be located mesially (see Fig. 13.23B, *3*; E, *10, 13,* and *16*) or distally (see Fig. 13.23B, *9*; E, *14*) on the root tip.

The distal canal may be slightly curved (see Fig. 13.23B, *1* to *5,* and *7*; E, *11, 14,* and *16*) or straight (see Fig. 13.23B, *4, 6, 8,* and *9*; E, *10, 12, 13, 17,* and *18*). The distal root may be slightly shorter than (see Fig. 13.23B, *1, 2, 4,* and *7*), equal to (see Fig. 13.23B, *3, 5,* and *6*; E, *10, 13, 14, 16,* and *17*), or longer than (see Fig. 13.23B, *8* and *9*; E, *11, 12, 15,* and *18*) the mesial root.

The distal canal is usually larger than the mesial canals (see Fig. 13.23B, *3, 4,* and *6* to *9*; E, *11, 13, 15,* and *16*) but may be equal to the mesial canals (see Fig. 13.23B, *1, 2,* and *5*; E, *12, 14,* and *18*). The distal canal tapers gently to the apex.

The apical foramen usually appears to be located at the tip of the root (see Fig. 13.23B, *1* to *7*; E, *10* to *13, 16,* and *18*), but the foramen may appear to exit mesially (see Fig. 13.23B, *9*) or distally (see Fig. 13.23B, *8*; E, *14, 15,* and *17*) to the apex of the root.

Cervical Cross Section (see Fig. 13.23C, 1 to 5)

The cervical cross section of the mandibular second molar is similar to that of the mandibular first molar (see Fig. 13.23C, *1* to *5*). The outline form of the mandibular second molar is more triangular (rather than quadrilateral, like that of the mandibular first molar) because of the smaller dimensions that are usually seen in the distal aspect of this tooth. The pulp chamber also tends to be triangular. The floor of the pulp chamber may have two openings, one mesially and one distally, which are centered within the dentin. If only one canal is present in the distal root, it will be centered within the dentin.

Midroot Cross Section (see Fig. 13.23C, 6 to 9)

Midroot cross sections of the mandibular molars demonstrate that the mesial root is very broad buccolingually and narrow mesiodistally (see Fig. 13.23C, *6* to *9*). The outline form is kidney-shaped (see Fig. 13.23C, *6* and *7*) or slightly in the form of a figure eight (see Fig. 13.23C, *8* and *9*).

The canals may be totally separate (see Fig. 13.23C, *9*) or confluent (see Fig. 13.23C, *6, 7,* and *8*), which makes it difficult to determine the presence of two mesial canals (see Fig. 13.23C, *8*). The distal root may be rounder than the mesial root because the outline form of this root is usually oval (see Fig. 13.23C, *6* and *9*);

however, broad distal roots are also seen (see Fig. 13.23C, *7* and *8*). One canal is usually present in the distal root, but two canals are often present.

Mandibular Third Molar

The pulp cavities of the mandibular third molar vary greatly (Fig. 13.24). The pulp cavity resembles the second mandibular molar most, but the crown looks too large for the roots, which may be shorter and curved and tend to be fused.

Buccolingual Section (see Fig. 13.24A and D)

In the buccolingual section, the pulp cavities of the mandibular third molar show a great deal of variation. Two roots and three canals are often present (see Fig. 13.24B, *6* and *7*), but two canals or two roots are also possible (see Fig. 13.24C, *8* and *9*). One canal and one root can also be found, but usually these teeth are not of much value for restorative purposes because they have short roots that taper quickly.

Most mandibular third molars have prominent pulp horns (see Fig. 13.24A, *1, 2,* and *4* to *9*; D, *10, 11, 12, 14, 15, 17,* and *18*), although others demonstrate small to nonexistent pulp horns (see Fig. 13.24A, *3*; D, *13* and *16*).

The mesial roots of most mandibular third molars (see Fig. 13.24A, *2* and *9*; D, *10, 11, 13,* and *14*) demonstrate a square pulp chamber (excluding the pulp horns). The mesial root usually has two canals (see Fig. 13.24A, *2, 5,* and *9*; D, *10, 11,* and *14*), but a single mesial root can be found (see Fig. 13.24D, *14*). The canals may be very curved (see Fig. 13.24A, *5* and *9*; D, *10*) or relatively straight (see Fig. 13.24A, *2*; D, *11* and *13*) as they taper gently toward the apical constriction.

The apical foramen usually appears to be located on the tip of the root (see Fig. 13.24A, *1* and *5*; D, *10, 11,* and *13*), but it may be located buccally (see Fig. 13.24A, *9*; D, *14*) or lingually to the tip of the root. If two canals are present, they usually possess separate apical foramina (see Fig. 13.24A, *2* and *5*; D, *10, 11,* and *13*), but some canals join in the apical region, exiting through a common foramen (see Fig. 13.24A, *9*).

The distal root of mandibular third molars possesses a very large pulp chamber and canal that are difficult to delineate into separate areas (see Fig. 13.24A, *1, 3, 4, 6, 7,* and *8*; D, *12,* and *15* to *18*).

The pulp canals, which are very large (see Fig. 13.24A, *1, 4, 6,* and *7*; D, *12, 15,* and *18*), may taper gently to the root tip (see Fig. 13.24A, *4, 6,* and *7*; D, *16* and *18*), or may demonstrate an abrupt constriction of the canal in the last few millimeters (see Fig. 13.24A, *1*; D, *12, 15,* and *17*).

The pulp chambers are square or rectangular (excluding the pulp horns). The pulp chambers, which are very small (see Fig. 13.24A, *3* and *8*), tend to show a constriction at the junction of the pulp chamber and canal, after which they taper gently to the apical constriction.

The apical foramen usually appears to be located at the tip of the root (see Fig. 13.24A, *3, 6, 7,* and *8*; D, *16* and *17*), but it may be located buccally or lingually to the root tip (see Fig. 13.24A, *1* and *4*; D, *15* and *18*).

Mesiodistal Section (see Fig. 13.24B and E)

The pulp horns of the mandibular third molar may be prominent (see Fig. 13.24B, *1* and *5*; E, *10, 11, 12, 14,* and *15*), small (see Fig. 13.24A, *4, 6,* and *7*; D, *17*), or nearly absent (see Fig. 13.24B, *2, 3, 8,* and *9*; E, *13, 16,* and *18*).

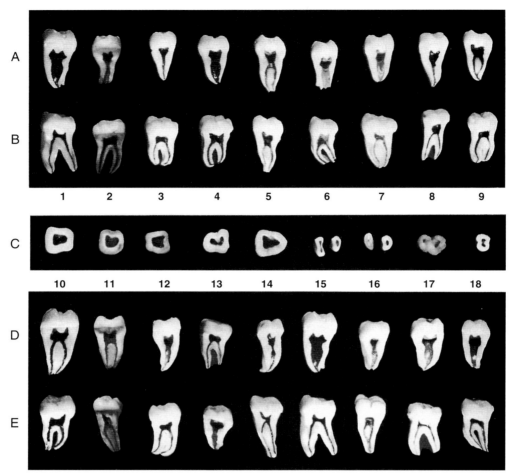

• **Fig. 13.24** Mandibular third molar. (A) Buccolingual section, exposing the mesial or distal aspect of the pulp cavity. This aspect does not appear on the dental radiographs. (B) Mesiodistal section, exposing the buccal or lingual aspect of the pulp cavity. (C) Five cross sections at the cervical line and four cross sections at the midroot. (D) Buccolingual section, exposing the mesial or distal aspect of the pulp cavity. (E) Mesiodistal section, exposing the buccal or lingual aspect of the pulp cavity.

The pulp chambers are usually square or rectangular (excluding pulp horns) when viewed from the buccal aspect (see Fig. 13.24B, *1* to *4*, *7*, and *9*; E, *10*, *12*, *13*, *15*, *17*, and *18*), but they may be somewhat square (see Fig. 13.24B, *5*; E, *14*).

The degree of curvature of the mesial root may be slight (see Fig. 13.24E, *13*, single-rooted), moderate (see Fig. 13.24B, *1, 2, 5, 8,* and *9*; E, *11, 15,* and *17*), or severe (see Fig. 13.24B, *3, 4, 6,* and *7*; E, *10, 12, 14, 16,* and *18*).

The canal within the mesial root may be large (see Fig. 13.24B, *2* and *4*; E, *10*) or very small (see Fig. 13.24B, *1, 3, 5, 8,* and *9*; E, *11, 12,* and *14* to *18*). The canals usually taper gently to the apical constriction. The apical foramen may appear to be located at the apex of the root (see Fig. 13.24B, *1, 2, 3, 5, 6, 8,* and *9*; E, *11, 12, 14, 17,* and *18*) or mesially (see Fig. 13.24B, *7*) or distally to the apex of the root (see Fig. 13.24B, *4*; E, *10* and *15*).

The length of the mesial roots may be equal to (see Fig. 13.24B, *2, 3,* and *8*; E, *10* and *11*), shorter than (see Fig. 13.24B, *5* and *9*; E, *18*), or longer than (see Fig. 13.24B, *1, 4, 6,* and *7*; E, *12, 14, 15,* and *17*) the length of the distal root.

The distal canal may be larger than the mesial canal (see Fig. 13.24B, *2* to *5* and *9*; E, *14* and *18*), but many are equal in size (see Fig. 13.24B, *1, 6, 7,* and *8*; E, *10, 11, 12, 15,* and *17*). The distal canal gently tapers to the apical constriction (see Fig. 13.24B, *1* to *8*; E, *10* to *18*).

The apical foramen may appear to be located at the apex of the root (see Fig. 13.24B, *1* to *5, 7,* and *9*; E, *10, 11, 12, 15, 17,* and *18*), or it may be mesial (see Fig. 13.24B, *8*) or distal (see Fig. 13.24B, *6*; E, *14*) to the apex of the root.

Some teeth show only one root with one or two canals. If only one canal is present (see Fig. 13.24E, *13*), the canal will be very large. If the third molar is multirooted, the canals will be much smaller (see Fig. 13.24E, *16*).

Cervical Cross Section (see Fig. 13.24C, 1 to 5)

The cervical cross section demonstrates a variable outline form that may be rectangular (see Fig. 13.24C, *1* to *4*) or triangular (see Fig. 13.24C, *5*).

Midroot Cross Section (see Fig. 13.24C, 6 to 9)

The mesial root, when present, is oval to figure eight in shape (see Fig. 13.24C, *6* and *7*). The distal root is oval (see Fig. 13.24C, *6*) or kidney-shaped (see Fig. 13.24C, *7*). If the roots are fused (see Fig. 13.24C, *8*) or only one root is present (see

Fig. 13.24C, *9*), the canals are usually larger. The canals in the roots that are kidney-shaped or are in the form of a figure eight are more ellipsoidal.

Radiographs: Pulp Chamber and Canals

Visualization of the pulp chamber and pulp canal or canals by standard radiography or digital radiography provides the clinician with evidence to augment what has been found clinically. All teeth should be examined periodically radiographically and clinically. Knowing what might be expected anatomically about the pulp chamber and pulp canals, which has been considered in a previous section, helps when radiographs are taken. The radiographs in Fig. 13.25, *A* through *I* illustrate normal pulp chambers and pulp canals. They are what are seen generally in the dental office, not the highly selected radiographs of the various teeth.

Crown and Root Fractures

Fractures of teeth may involve the crown, the crown and root, or the root. Probably the most common are fractures of the crown. In some cracked teeth, only the enamel is involved; in others, both the enamel and dentin may be affected; but initially or later, the pulp also may be involved with or without the loss of tooth structure (e.g., cusp). In severe trauma, the whole crown may be lost. The clinician should be familiar with the most likely places, morphologically, for cracking or fractures to occur. The most likely places involve developmental grooves (Fig 13.26), often in relation to restorations.

Fractures of cusps of the maxillary first premolar and mandibular first molars often occur along developmental grooves or stress lines, as shown in Fig. 13.26. Such fractures may occur in connection with bruxism and clenching. It is not uncommon for the distolingual cusp of the mandibular first molar to fracture in association with a large restoration, which leads to pulpitis (Fig. 13.27).

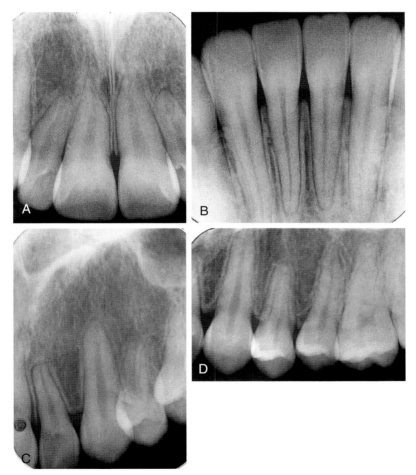

• **Fig. 13.25** (A) Large pulp chambers and pulp canals in a young adult. (B) Mandibular incisors. Normal pulp canals. (C) Lateral incisor and canine. Normal chambers and canals. Root resorption on lateral incisor. (D) Maxillary canine and premolars with normal chambers and canals. Root resorption on first premolar associated with orthodontics. (E) Mandibular lateral incisor, canine, and first premolar with normal chambers and canals. (F) Mandibular second premolar and first and second molars with normal chambers and canals. Note curvature of the mesial root of the first molar. (G) Mandibular molars and premolars with normal chambers and pulp canals. (H) Impacted third molar adjacent to second mandibular molar. The pulp chambers and pulp canals are normal. (I) First and second primary molars being resorbed in association with the erupting permanent premolars. Mandibular second molar in the process of erupting.

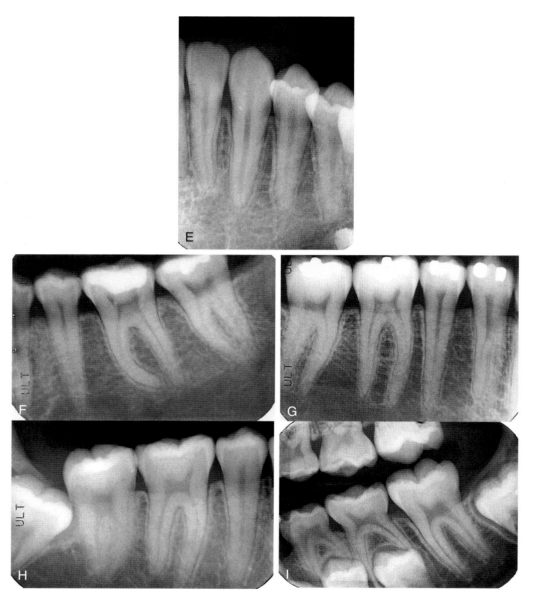

Fig. 13.25, cont'd

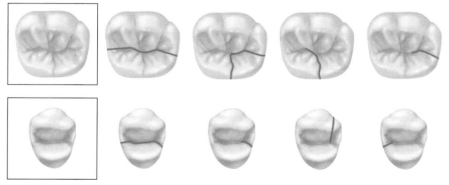

• **Fig. 13.26** Fracture lines most commonly seen in the first maxillary premolar and first mandibular molar.

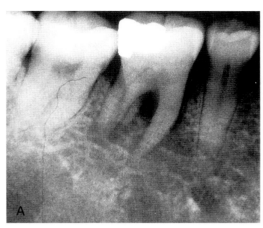
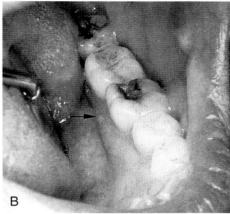

• **Fig. 13.27** (A) Radiograph showing periapical radiolucency associated with parulis shown in (B). (B) Fracture of distolingual cusp related to undermined tooth structure and amalgam restoration. (From Ash MM, Ramjford S: *Occlusion,* ed 4, Philadelphia, 1995, Saunders.)

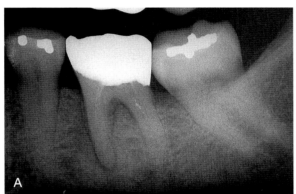

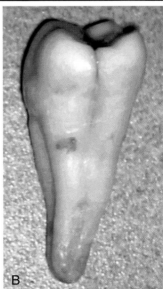

• **Fig. 13.28** (A) Radiograph showing loss of lamina dura on the mesial root of the mandibular molar but no indication of root fracture. (B) Longitudinal fracture on the distal aspect of the crown and coronal root. (A, From Ash MM: *Schienentherapie,* ed 2, Munich, 1999, Urban & Fischer; B, from Cohen S, Hargreaves KM: *Pathways of the pulp*, ed 9, St Louis, 2006, Mosby.)

Fractures of the root cause symptoms that resemble those of other dental problems; therefore the diagnosis of root fracture may be difficult,[4] especially when the fracture does not appear on the radiograph (Fig. 13.28).

Fractures may extend from the crown and may reach the pulp or involve only the root adjacent to the periodontal ligament. Horizontal root fractures are most likely the result of external physical trauma or clenching and bruxism. Vertical root fractures may be caused by bruxing and clenching or may be the result of restorations with endodontic posts in root canals.

Relation of Posterior Root Apices to the Mandibular Canal

Of interest to the clinician doing endodontics, periapical surgery, or placement of implants is the position of the mandibular nerve (canal) and the mental foramen.

The mandibular nerve traversing the mandible in the mandibular canal occupies different positions relative to the apices of the molar and premolar teeth (Fig. 13.29, *A to D*). In Fig. 13.30, the distances from the outer to the inner surface of the buccal plate *(1)*, from the inner surface of the cortical plate to the apex of a tooth *(2)*, and from the canal to the apex of the tooth *(3)* reflect the data obtained from sections of the mandible.[5]

The mean width of the buccal plate (see Fig. 13.30B, *1*) over the premolar is 1.9 ± 0.49 mm; over the first molar, 2.38 ± 0.57 mm; over the second molar, 5.6 ± 0.93 mm; and over the third molar, 2.34 ± 1.0 mm.

The mean distance from the inner buccal plate to the apex of the tooth (see Fig. 13.30B, *2*) for the second premolar is 3.78 ± 1.04 mm; for the first molar, 4.1 ± 0.98 mm; for the second molar, 7.1 ± 1.4 mm; and for the third molar, 4.03 ± 1.8 mm.

The mean vertical distance from the canal to the apex (see Fig. 13.30B, *3*) for the second premolar is 3.07 ± 0.43 mm; for the first molar, 4.03 ± 0.31 mm; for the second molar, 2.5 ± 0.25 mm; and for the third molar, 1.96 ± 0.27 mm.

With regard to the buccolingual alignment of the mandibular canal to root apices, the canal is in vertical alignment with the second premolars for 65% of the time, slightly lingual to the apices of the first molar apices for 71% of the time, in line with the apices of second molars for 73% of the time, and in line with the third molars for 56% of the time.

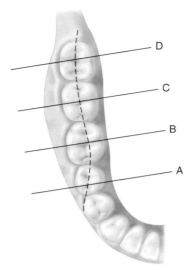

• **Fig. 13.29** Diagrammatic representation of sections through the mandible at the position of the second premolar and first, second, and third molars. Dotted line represents the faciolingual position of the mandibular canal.

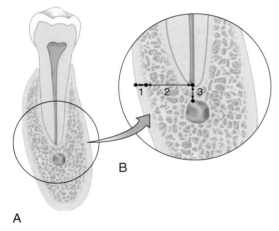

• **Fig. 13.30** (A) Diagrammatic representation of a cross section of the mandible. (B) Enlarged view with three measurements taken as indicated in the text.

Data are based on the vertical axis of each tooth with the recognition that more than one apex is present. Thus the position of the mandibular canal relative to the apices of the teeth tends to follow the dotted line in Fig. 13.29.

The position of the mental foramen relative to the mandibular premolars and first molar can be described as follows: the foramen is between the first and second premolars 33% of the time, in line with the second premolar 11% of the time, and distal to the second premolar 56% of the time. In terms of vertical position, the foramen can be found coronal to the apices 22% of the time, at the apices 15% of the time, and below the apices 63% of the time.[5]

Pretest Answers

1. A
2. A
3. C
4. D
5. D

References

1. Kronfeld R: *Dental histology and comparative dental anatomy*, Philadelphia, 1937, Lea & Febiger.
2. Riethmuller RH: The filling of root canals with Prinz' paraffin compound, *Dent Cosmos* 56:490, 1914.
3. Ahmed HA, Abu-bakr NH, Yahia HA, Ibrahim YE: Root and canal morphology of permanent mandibular molars in a Sudanese population, *Int End J* 40:766–771, 2007.
4. Mullally BH, Ahmed M: Periodontal signs and symptoms associated with vertical root fracture, *Dent Update* 27:356, 2000.
5. Ash JL, Ash CM: Mandibular canal and mental foramen: relation to posterior root apices, *J Dent Res* 1997. (Abstract).

Bibliography

Acosta Vigouroux AS, et al.: Anatomy of the pulp chamber floor of the permanent maxillary first molar, *J Endod* 4:214, 1978.

Barker BC, et al.: Anatomy of root canals: I. Permanent incisors, canines and premolars, *Aust Dent J* 18:320, 1973.

Barker BC, et al.: Anatomy of root canals. II. Permanent maxillary molars, *Aust Dent J* 19:46, 1974.

Barker, B. C., et al. Anatomy of root canals. III. Permanent mandibular molars. *Aust Dent J* 19:408, 1974.

Burah JG, et al.: A study of the presence of accessory foramina and the topography of molar furcations, *Oral Surg* 38:451, 1974.

Carlsen O, Andersen J: On the anatomy of the pulp chamber and root canals in human deciduous teeth, *Tandlaegebladet* 70:93, 1966.

Carlsen O, Andersen J: Radix mesiolingualis and radix distolingualis in a collection of permanent maxillary molars, *Acta Odontol Scand* 58:229, 2000.

Carlsen O, Andersen J: Radix paramolaris and distomolaris in Danish permanent maxillary molars, *Acta Odontol Scand* 57:283, 1999.

Carns EJ, Skidmore AE: Configurations and deviations of root canals of maxillary first premolars, *Oral Surg* 36:880, 1973.

Gardner DG, et al.: Taurodontism, shovel-shaped incisors and the Klinefelter syndrome, *Dent J* 44:372, 1980. 1978.

Harris, WE. Unusual root canal anatomy in the maxillary molar. *J Endod* 6,573, 1980.

Hess W, Zurcher E: *The anatomy of root canals*, London, 1925, John Bale Sons and Danielsson.

Ibrahim SM, et al.: Pulp cavities of permanent teeth, *Egypt Dent J* 23:83, 1977.

Kerekes K, et al.: Morphometric observations on the root canals of human molars, *J Endod* 3:114, 1977.

Kirkham DB: The location and incidence of accessory pulp canals in periodontal pockets, *J Am Dent Assoc* 91:353, 1975.

Mageean JF: The significance of root canal morphology in endodontics, *J Br Endod Soc* 6:67, 1972.

Middletoti-Shaw JC: *The teeth, the bony palate and the mandible in Bantu races of South Africa*, London, 1931, John Bale Sons and Danielsson.

Okumura T: Anatomy of the root canals, *J Am Dent Assoc* 14:632, 1927.

Senyurek MS: Pulp cavities of molars in primates, *Am J Phys Anthropol* 25:119, 1939.

Stone LH, et al.: Maxillary molars demonstrating more than one palatal root canal, *Oral Surg* 51:649, 1981.

Sutalo J, et al.: Morphologic characteristics of root canals in upper and lower premolars, *Acta Stomatol Croat* 14:23, 1980.

Tidmarsh BG: Micromorphology of pulp chambers in human molar teeth, *Int Endod J* 13:69, 1980.

Vertucci FJ, Williams RG: Furcation canals in the human mandibular first molar, *Oral Surg* 38:308, 1974.

Vertucci FJ, et al.: Root canal morphology of the human maxillary first premolar, *Oral Surg* 99:194, 1979.

Vertucci FJ, et al.: Root canal morphology of the human maxillary second premolar, *Oral Surg* 88:456, 1974.

Warren EM: The relationship between crown size and the incidence of bifid root canals in mandibular incisor teeth, *Oral Surg* 52:425, 1981.

Dento-Osseous Structures, Blood Vessels, and Nerves

LEARNING OBJECTIVES

1. Correctly define and pronounce the new terms as emphasized in the bold type.
2. Identify the primary bony landmarks of the maxilla and the mandible.
3. Describe the form of the alveoli for each permanent tooth.
4. List the arterial supply for each permanent tooth
5. List the nerve supply to the jaws and teeth.

Pretest Questions

1. The area of the superior border of the ramus between the condyle and coronoid process is known as which of the following?
   A. Pterygoid fovea
   B. Mandibular notch
   C. Coronoid notch
   D. Temporomandibular joint
2. The ridge of the maxilla overlying the maxillary canine is also known as which of the following?
   A. Canine ridge
   B. Canine eminence
   C. Canine bulge
   D. Canine fossa
3. The most posterior and inferior aspect of the maxilla is a prominent area that overlies the root of the third molar. Which of the following is the name given to this portion of the maxilla?
   A. Palatine process
   B. Lateral pterygoid plate
   C. Maxillary tuberosity
   D. Zygomatic process of the maxilla
4. The ridge where the two halves of the mandible are joined/fused shortly after birth at the median line is referred to as which of the following?
   A. Symphysis
   B. Mental tubercle
   C. Genial tubercle
   D. Ramus
5. The lingula provides attachment for which of the following structures?
   A. Stylomandibular ligament
   B. Medial pterygoid muscle
   C. Sphenomandibular ligament
   D. Lateral pterygoid muscle

For additional study resources, please visit Expert Consult.

The development of the dentitions has been discussed and a brief review of the development of the neurocranium and splanchnocranium has been presented in Chapter 2. Therefore, in this chapter, the focus is on the dentoalveolar and dento-osseous structures of the permanent dentition. The forms of the roots of the teeth and their sizes and angulations govern the shape of the alveoli in the jawbones, and this in turn shapes the contour of the dento-osseous portions facially.

The osseous structures that support the teeth are the maxilla and the mandible. The maxilla, or upper jaw, consists of two bones: a right maxilla and a left maxilla sutured together at the median line. Both maxillae in turn are joined to other bones of the head (Fig. 14.1). The mandible, or lower jaw, has no osseous union with the skull and is a movable (ginglymoarthrodial) joint.

The Maxillae

The maxillae make up a large part of the bony framework of the facial portion of the skull. They form the major portion of the roof of the mouth, or hard palate, and assist in the formation of the floor of the orbit and the sides and base of the nasal cavity. They support the 16 permanent maxillary teeth.

Each maxilla is an irregular bone, somewhat cuboidal in shape, which consists of a body and four processes: the zygomatic, frontal, palatine, and alveolar processes. The maxilla is hollow and contains the maxillary sinus air space, also called the **antrum of Highmore**. From the dental viewpoint, in addition to its general shape and the processes mentioned, several landmarks on this bone are among the most important, including the incisive fossa, canine fossa, canine eminence, infraorbital foramen, posterior alveolar foramina, maxillary tuberosity, pterygopalatine fossa, and incisive canal.

The body of the maxilla has the following four surfaces: anterior or facial, infratemporal, orbital, and nasal.

Anterior Surface

The anterior or facial surface (Figs. 14.2 and 14.3) is separated above from the orbital aspect by the infraorbital ridge. Medially, it is limited by the margin of the nasal notch, and posteriorly, it is separated from the posterior surface by the anterior border of the zygomatic process, which has a confluent ridge directly over the roots of the first molar. The ridge corresponding to the root of the canine tooth is usually the most pronounced and is called the **canine eminence**.

Anterior to the canine eminence, overlying the roots of the incisor teeth, is a shallow concavity known as the **incisive fossa**.

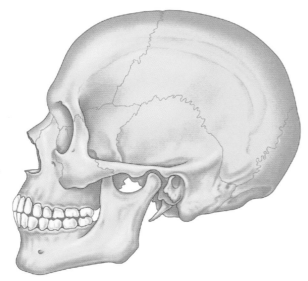

• **Fig. 14.1** Representation of an adult skull with permanent dentition. The maxilla consists of a body and four processes (malar, nasal, alveolar, and palatine) that articulate by synarthrosis with cranial and other facial bones (e.g., frontal, nasal, ethmoid, malar bones). The mandible articulates with the temporal bone by the temporomandibular joint (see Fig. 15.6).

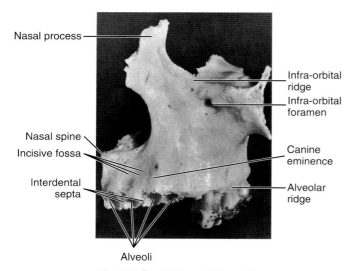

• **Fig. 14.2** Frontal view of left maxilla.

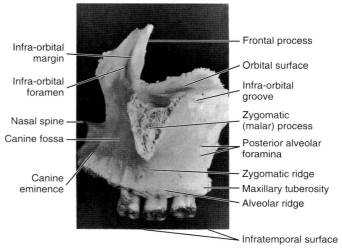

• **Fig. 14.3** Lateral view of left maxilla.

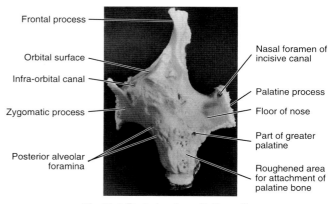

• **Fig. 14.4** Posterior view of left maxilla.

Posterior to the canine eminence on a higher level is a deeper concavity called the **canine fossa**. The floor of this canine fossa is formed in part by the projecting zygomatic process. Above this fossa and below the infraorbital ridge is the infraorbital foramen, the external opening of the infraorbital canal. The major portion of the canine fossa is directly above the roots of the premolars.

Posterior Surface

The posterior or infratemporal surface (Fig. 14.4; see also Fig. 14.3) is bounded above by the posterior edge of the orbital surface. Inferiorly and anteriorly, it is separated from the anterior surface by the zygomatic process and the zygomatic ridge, which runs from the inferior border of the zygomatic process to the alveolus of the maxillary first molar. This surface is more or less convex and is pierced in a downward direction by two or more posterior alveolar foramina. These two canals are on a level with the lower border of the zygomatic process and are somewhat distal to the roots of the third molar.

The inferior portion of this surface is more prominent where it overhangs the root of the third molar and is called the **maxillary tuberosity**. Medially, this tuberosity is limited by a sharp, irregular margin that articulates with the pyramidal process of the palatine bone and, in some cases, the lateral pterygoid plate of the sphenoid bone. The maxillary tuberosity is the origin for some fibers of the medial pterygoid muscle.

A portion of the infratemporal surface superior to the maxillary tuberosity is the anterior boundary to the pterygomaxillary fissure.

Orbital Surface

The orbital surface is smooth and together with the orbital surface of the zygomatic bone forms the floor of the orbit. The junction of this surface and the anterior surface forms the infraorbital margin or ridge, which runs superiorly to form part of the nasal process. Its posterior border or edge coincides with the inferior boundary of the inferior orbital fissure.

The thin medial edge of the orbital surface is notched anteriorly, forming the lacrimal groove. Behind this groove, it articulates for a short distance with the lacrimal bone, then for a greater length with a thin portion of the ethmoid bone, and terminates posteriorly in a surface that articulates with the orbital process of the palatal bone. Its lateral area is continuous with the base of the zygomatic process (see Fig. 14.3).

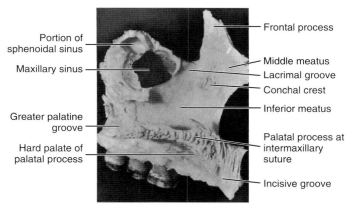

• **Fig. 14.5** Medial view of left maxilla.

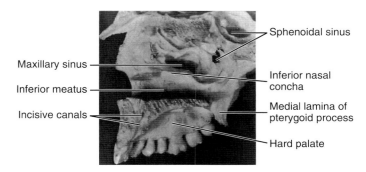

• **Fig. 14.6** Medial view of right maxilla. This specimen has not been disarticulated completely and has the maxillary teeth in situ.

Traversing the posterior portion of the orbital surface is the infraorbital groove. This groove begins at the center of the posterior surface and runs anteriorly. The anterior portion of this groove is covered, becoming the infraorbital canal, the anterior opening of which is located directly below the infraorbital ridge on the anterior surface.

If the covered portion of this canal were to be laid open, the orifices of the middle and anterior superior alveolar canal would be seen transmitting the corresponding vessels and nerves to the premolars, canines, and incisor teeth.

Nasal Surface

The nasal surface (Figs. 14.5 and 14.6) is directed medially toward the nasal cavity. It is bordered below by the superior surface of the palatine process. Anteriorly, it is limited by the sharp edge of the nasal notch. Above and anteriorly, it is continuous with the medial surface of the frontal process. Behind this, it is deeply channeled by the lacrimal groove, which is converted into a canal by articulation with the lacrimal and inferior turbinate bones.

Behind this groove, the upper edge of the nasal surface corresponds to the medial margin of the orbital surface, and the maxilla articulates in this region with the lacrimal bone, a thin portion of the ethmoid bone, and the orbital process of the palatine bone.

The posterior border of the maxilla, which articulates with the palatine bone, is traversed obliquely from above downward and slightly medially by a groove, which, by articulation with the palate bone, is converted into the greater palatine canal. Toward the posterior and upper part of this nasal surface, a large, irregular opening into the maxillary sinus (antrum of Highmore) may be seen. In an articulated skull, this opening is partially covered by the uncinate process of the ethmoid bone and the inferior nasal concha.

Anterior to the lacrimal groove, the nasal surface is ridged for the attachment of the inferior nasal concha. Below this, the bone forms a lateral wall of the inferior nasal meatus. Above the ridge for a small distance on the medial side of the nasal process, the smooth lateral wall of the middle meatus appears.

Zygomatic Process

The zygomatic process may be seen in the lateral views of the maxillary bone as a roughly triangular eminence whose apex is placed inferiorly directly over the first molar roots. The lateral border is rough and sponge-like in appearance, where it has been disarticulated from the zygomatic or cheek bone (see Figs. 14.1 and 14.3).

Frontal Process

The frontal process (see Figs. 14.2 to 14.5) arises from the upper and anterior body of the maxilla.

Part of this process is formed by the upward continuation of the infraorbital margin medially. Its edge articulates with the nasal bone. Superiorly, the process articulates with the frontal bone. The medial surface of the frontal process forms part of the lateral wall of the nasal cavity. Anteriorly, the frontal process articulates with the nasal bone.

Palatine Process

The palatine process (see Figs. 14.2 to 14.8) is a horizontal ledge extending medially from the nasal surface of the maxilla. Its superior surface forms a major portion of the nasal floor. The inferior surfaces of the combined left and right palatine processes form the hard palate as far posteriorly as the second molar, where they articulate with the horizontal parts of the palatine bone (Figs. 14.7 and 14.8) at the transverse palatine suture.

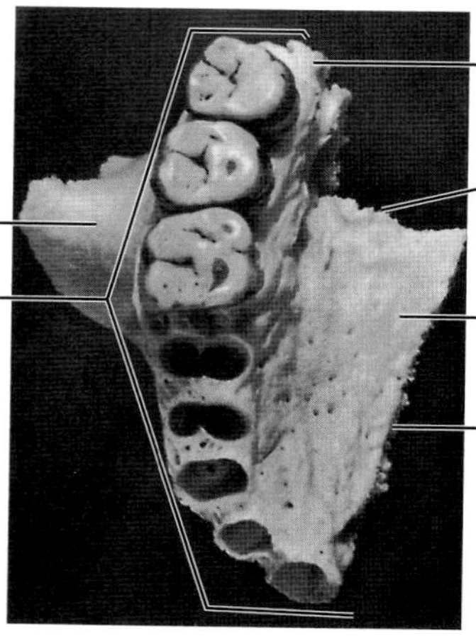

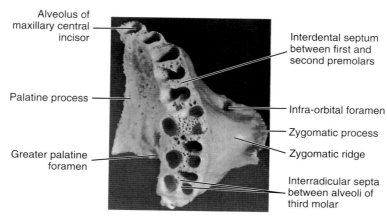

• **Fig. 14.7** Palatine view of maxilla. Note the dental foramina in the deepest portion of the permanent first molar alveolus.

• **Fig. 14.8** View of inferior surface of the maxilla showing alveolar process and alveoli.

The inferior surface of the palatine process is rough and pitted for the palatine mucous glands in the roof of the mouth and is pierced by numerous small foramina for the passage of blood vessels and nerve fibers. At the posterior border of the process is a groove or canal that passes the greater palatine nerve and vessels to the palatal soft tissues. The posterior edge of the palatine process becomes relatively thin where it joins the palatine bone at the point of the greater palatine foramen. The palatine process becomes progressively thicker anteriorly from the posterior border. Anteriorly, the palatal process is confluent with the alveolar process surrounding the roots of the anterior teeth.

Immediately posterior to the central incisor alveolus, when looking at the medial aspect of the maxilla, one sees a smooth groove that is half of the incisive canal, when the two maxillae are joined together. The incisive fossa into which the canals open may be seen immediately lingual to the central incisors at the median line, or intermaxillary suture where the maxillae are joined. Two canals open laterally into the incisive foramen, the foramina of Stenson, carrying the nasopalatine nerves and vessels.

Occasionally, two midline foramina are present, the foramina of Scarpi.

Extending laterally from the incisive foramen to the space between the lateral incisor and canine alveoli are the remnants of the suture between the maxilla and premaxilla. In most mammals, the premaxilla remains an independent bone.

Alveolar Process

The alveolar process makes up the inferior portion of the maxilla; it is the portion of the bone that surrounds the roots of the maxillary teeth and that gives them their osseous support. The process extends from the base of the tuberosity posterior to the last molar to the median line anteriorly, where it articulates with the same process of the opposite maxilla (see Figs. 14.7 and 14.8). It merges with the palatine process medially and with the zygomatic process laterally (see Fig. 14.8).

When one looks directly at the inferior aspect of the maxilla toward the alveoli with the teeth removed, it is apparent that the alveolar process is curved to conform with the dental arch. It completes, with its fellow of the opposite side, the alveolar arch supporting the roots of the teeth of the maxilla.

The process has a facial (labial and buccal) surface and a lingual surface with ridges corresponding to the surfaces of the roots of the teeth supported by it. It is made up of labiobuccal and lingual plates of very dense but thin cortical bone separated by interdental septa of cancellous bone.

The facial plate is thin, and the positions of the alveoli are well marked on it by visible ridges as far posteriorly as the distobuccal root of the first molar (see Fig. 14.2). The margins of these alveoli are frail, and their edges are sharp and thin. The buccal plate over the second and third molars, including the alveolar margins, is thicker. In general, the lingual plate of the alveolar process is heavier than the facial plate. In addition, the alveolar process is longer where it surrounds the anterior teeth, sometimes extending posteriorly to include the premolars. In short, it extends farther down in covering the lingual portion of the roots.

The bone is very thick lingually over the deeper portions of the alveoli of the anterior teeth and premolars. The merging of the alveolar process with the palatal process brings about this formation. The lingual plate is paper thin over the lingual alveolus of the first molar, however, and rather thin over the lingual alveoli of the second and third molars. This thin lingual plate over the molar roots is part of the formation of the greater palatine canal (see Fig. 14.8).

The alveolar process is maintained by the presence of the teeth. Should any tooth be lost, the portion of the alveolar process that supported the missing tooth will be subject to atrophic reduction. Should all the teeth be lost, the alveolar process will eventually be virtually lost.

Alveoli (Tooth Sockets)

The alveolar cavities are formed by the facial and lingual plates of the alveolar process and by connecting septa of bone placed between the two plates. The form and depth of each alveolus are determined by the form and length of the root it supports (see Table 1.1).

The alveolus nearest the median line is that of the central incisor (Fig. 14.9; see also Fig. 14.8). The periphery is regular and round, and the interior of the alveolus is evenly tapered and triangular in cross section, with the apex toward the lingual.

The second alveolus in line is that of the lateral incisor. It is generally conical and egg-shaped, or ovoid, with the widest portion to the labial. It is narrower mesiodistally than labiolingually and is smaller on cross section, although it is often deeper than the central alveolus. Sometimes it is curved at the upper extremity (Fig. 14.10; see also Fig. 14.8).

The canine alveolus is the third from the median line. It is much larger and deeper than those just described. The periphery is oval and regular in outline, with the labial width greater than the lingual. The socket extends distally. It is flattened mesially and somewhat concave distally. The bone is so frail at the canine eminence on the facial surface of the alveolus that the root of the canine is often exposed on the labial surface near the middle third (see Fig. 14.2).

The first premolar alveolus (see Figs. 14.8 and 14.10) is kidney-shaped in cross section, with the cavity partially divided by a spine of bone that fits into the mesial developmental groove of the root of this tooth. This spine divides the cavity into a buccal and a lingual portion. If the tooth root is bifurcated for part of its length,

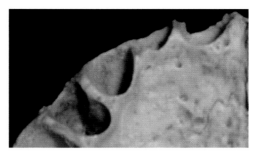

• **Fig. 14.9** Alveoli of the central incisor, lateral incisor, and canine. (Case and photographs courtesy Lawrence C. Zoller, PhD, Las Vegas, NV.)

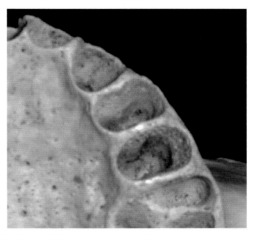

• **Fig. 14.10** Alveoli of the premolar area. (Case and photographs courtesy Lawrence C. Zoller, PhD, Las Vegas, NV.)

as is often the case, the terminal portion of the cavity is separated into buccal and lingual alveoli. The socket is flattened distally and much wider buccolingually than mesiodistally (see Table 1.1).

The second premolar alveolus is also kidney-shaped, but the curvatures are in reverse to those of the first premolar alveolus. The proportions and depth are almost the same. The septal spine is located on the distal side instead of the medial side, because the second premolar root is inclined to have a well-defined developmental groove distally. This tooth usually has one broad root with a blunt end, but it is occasionally bifurcated at the apical third.

The first molar alveolus (see Figs. 14.8 and 14.11) is made up of three distinct alveoli widely separated. The lingual alveolus is the largest; it is round, regular, and deep. The cavity extends in the direction of the hard palate, having a lingual plate over it that is very thin. The lingual periphery of this alveolus is extremely sharp and frail. This condition may contribute to the tissue recession often seen at this site.

The mesiobuccal and distobuccal alveoli of the first molar have no outstanding characteristics except that the buccal plates are thin. The bone is somewhat thicker at the peripheries than that found on the lingual alveolus. Nevertheless, it is thinner farther up on the buccal plate. It is not uncommon for one to find the roots uncovered by bone in spots when examining dry specimens.

The forms of the buccal alveoli resemble the forms of the roots they support. The mesiobuccal alveolus is broad buccolingually, with the mesial and distal walls flattened. The distobuccal alveolus is rounder and more conical.

The septa that separate the three alveoli (interradicular septa) are broad at the area that corresponds to the root bifurcation, and they become progressively thicker as the peripheries of the alveoli are approached. The bone septa are very cancellous, which denotes a rich blood supply, as is true of all the septa, including those separating the various teeth as well.

A general description of the alveoli of the second molar would coincide with that of the first molar; these alveoli are closer together, since the roots of this tooth do not spread as much. As a consequence, the septa separating the alveoli are not as heavy.

The third molar alveolus is similar to that of the second molar, except that it is somewhat smaller in all dimensions. Fig. 14.11 shows a third molar socket to accommodate a tooth with three well-defined roots, a rare occurrence. Usually, the two buccal (and often all three) roots will be fused. The interradicular septum changes accordingly. If the roots of the tooth are fused, a septal spine will appear in the alveolus at the points of fusion on the roots marked by deep developmental grooves.

Maxillary Sinus

The maxillary sinus lies within the body of the bone and is of corresponding pyramidal form; the base is directed toward the nasal cavity. Its summit extends laterally into the root of the zygomatic process. It is closed in laterally and above by the thin walls that form the anterolateral, posterolateral, and orbital surfaces of the body. The sinus overlies the alveolar process in which the molar teeth are implanted, more particularly, the first and second molars, the alveoli of which are separated from the sinus by a thin layer of bone. Occasionally, the maxillary sinus will extend forward far enough to overlie the premolars also. It is not uncommon to find the bone covering the alveoli of some of the posterior teeth extending above the floor of the cavity of the maxillary sinus, forming small hillocks.

Regardless of the irregularity and the extension of the alveoli into the maxillary sinus, a layer of bone always separates the roots of the teeth and the floor of the sinus in the absence of pathological conditions. A layer of sinus mucosa is also always between the root tips and the sinus cavity.

Maxillary Articulation

The maxilla articulates with the nasal, frontal, lacrimal, and ethmoid bones, above and laterally with the zygomatic bone, and occasionally with the sphenoid bone. Posteriorly and medially, it articulates with the palatal bone. Medially, it supports the inferior turbinate and the vomer and articulates with the opposite maxilla.

The Mandible

The mandible (Figs. 14.12 to 14.23) is horseshoe-shaped and supports the teeth of the lower dental arch. This bone is movable and has no bony articulation with the skull. It is the heaviest and strongest bone of the head and serves as a framework for the floor of the mouth. It is situated immediately below the maxillary and zygomatic bone, and its condyles rest in the mandibular fossa of the temporal bone. This articulation is the temporomandibular joint.

The mandible has a horizontal portion, or body, and two vertical portions, or rami. The rami join the body at an obtuse angle.

The body consists of two lateral halves, which are joined at the median line shortly after birth. The line of fusion, usually marked by a slight ridge, is called the **symphysis.** The body of the mandible has two surfaces (one external and one internal) and two borders (one superior and one inferior).

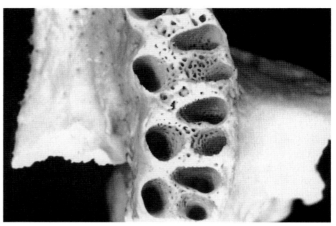

• **Fig. 14.11** Alveoli of the molar area. Note the thinness of the buccal plates over the first molar roots compared with those of the second and third maxillary molars. The third molar alveoli are rarely separated as distinctly as seen in this specimen. Figs. 14.9 to 14.11 demonstrate a number of significant points concerning the maxillary alveoli. In Fig. 14.9, the facial cortical plate of bone is thin over the anterior teeth and is considerably thicker over the posterior teeth, especially the molars. Cancellous bone seems to exist buccal to some of the posterior roots. In Fig. 14.10, interradicular septa are thick but with numerous nutrient canals. In Fig. 14.11, cancellous bone, furnishing numerous opportunities for blood supply, is evident in the apical portions of the alveoli. The anterior alveoli are lined laterally with a layer of smooth cortical bone. This lining is less prominent in the posterior alveoli.

To the right and left of the symphysis, near the lower border of the mandible, are two prominences called **mental tubercles**. A prominent triangular surface made by the symphysis and these two tubercles is called the **mental protuberance** (see Fig. 14.16).

Immediately posterior to the symphysis and immediately above the mental protuberance is a shallow depression called the incisive fossa. The fossa is immediately below the alveolar border of the central and lateral incisors and anterior to the canines. The alveolar portion of the mandible overlying the root of the canine is prominent and is called the canine eminence of the mandible. However, this eminence does not extend down very far toward the lower border of the mandible before it is lost in the prominence of the mental protuberance and the lower border of the mandible.

The external surface of the mandible from a lateral viewpoint presents a number of important areas for examination.

The **oblique ridge** (oblique line, radiographically) extends obliquely across the external surface of the mandible from the mental tubercle to the anterior border of the ramus, with which it is continuous. It lies below the mental foramen. It is usually not prominent except in the molar area (see Fig. 14.12).

This ridge thins out as it progresses upward and becomes the anterior border of the ramus and ends at the tip of the **coronoid process**. The coronoid process is one of two processes making up the superior border of the ramus. It is a pointed, flattened, smooth projection and is roughened toward the tip to give attachment for a part of the temporal muscle.

The **condyle**, or **condyloid process**, on the posterior border of the ramus is variable in form. It is divided into a superior or articular portion and an inferior portion, or neck. Although the articular portion, the condyle, appears as a rounded knob when the mandible is viewed from a lateral aspect, from a posterior aspect, the condyle is much wider and oblong in outline (compare Figs. 14.12 and 14.13).

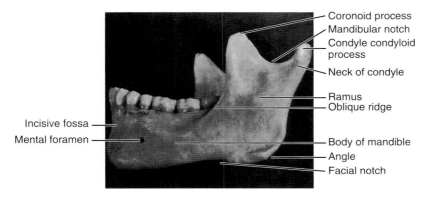

Coronoid process
Mandibular notch
Condyle condyloid process
Neck of condyle
Ramus
Oblique ridge
Incisive fossa
Mental foramen
Body of mandible
Angle
Facial notch

• **Fig. 14.12** View of outer surface of mandible.

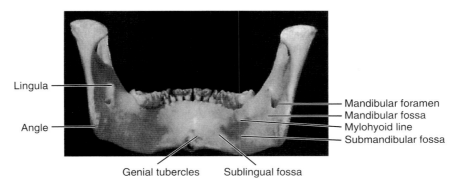

Lingula
Angle
Mandibular foramen
Mandibular fossa
Mylohyoid line
Submandibular fossa
Genial tubercles   Sublingual fossa

• **Fig. 14.13** Posterior view of mandible.

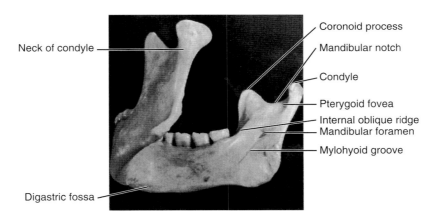

Neck of condyle
Coronoid process
Mandibular notch
Condyle
Pterygoid fovea
Internal oblique ridge
Mandibular foramen
Mylohyoid groove
Digastric fossa

• **Fig. 14.14** Posterolateral view of medial surface of mandible.

The condyle is convex, fitting into the mandibular fossa of the temporal bone when the mandible is articulated to the skull, and forms, with the interarticular cartilage that lies between the two surfaces and with the tissue attachment, the temporomandibular joint (see Fig. 15.2).

The neck of the condyle is a constricted portion immediately below the articular surface. It is flattened in front and presents a concave pit medially, the **pterygoid fovea**. A smooth, semicircular notch, the **mandibular notch**, forms the sharp upper border of the ramus between the condyle and coronoid process (see Fig. 14.14).

The distal border of the ramus is smooth and rounded and presents a concave outline from the neck of the condyle to the angle of the jaw, where the posterior border of the ramus and the inferior border of the body of the mandible join. The border of

this angle is rough, being the attachment of the masseter muscle (see Fig. 15.18) and the stylomandibular ligament (see Fig. 15.7).

An important landmark on the lateral aspect of the mandible is the **mental foramen**. It should be noted that this opening of the anterior end of the mandibular canal is directed upward, backward, and laterally. The foramen is usually located midway between the superior and inferior border of the body of the mandible when the teeth are in position, and most often, it is below the second premolar tooth, a little below the apex of the root. The position of this foramen is not constant, and it may be between the first premolar and the second premolar tooth. After the teeth are lost and resorption of alveolar bone has taken place, the mental foramen may appear near the crest of the alveolar border. In childhood, before the first permanent molar has come into position, this foramen is usually immediately below the first primary molar and nearer to the lower border.

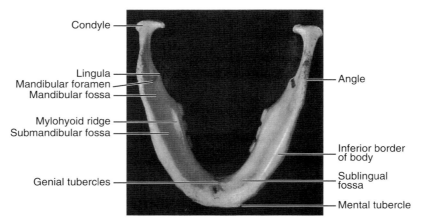

• **Fig. 14.15** View of mandible from below.

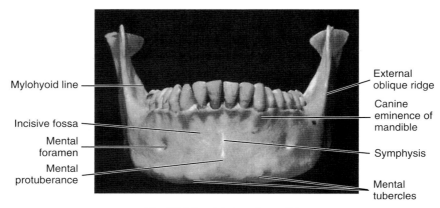

• **Fig. 14.16** Frontal view of mandible.

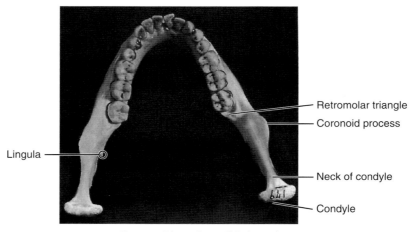

• **Fig. 14.17** View of mandible from above.

It is interesting to note that when the mandible is observed from a point directly opposite the first molar, most of the distal half of the third molar is hidden by the anterior border of the ramus. When the mandible is viewed from in front, directly opposite the median line, the second and third molars are located 5 to 7 mm lingually to the anterior border of the ramus (compare Figs. 14.12 and 14.16).

Internal Surface of the Mandible

Observation of the mandible from the rear shows that the median line is marked by a slight vertical depression, representing the line of union of the right and left halves of the mandible, and that immediately below this, at the lower third, the bone is roughened by eminences called the **superior** and **inferior mental spines**, or genial tubercles (see Figs. 14.15 and 14.34C).

The internal surface of the body of the mandible is divided into two portions by a well-defined ridge: the **mylohyoid line**. It occupies a position closely corresponding to the lateral oblique ridge on the surface. It starts at or near the lowest part of the mental spines and passes backward and upward, increasing in prominence until the anterior portion of the ramus is reached; there, it smooths out and gradually disappears (see Figs. 14.14 and 14.34C).

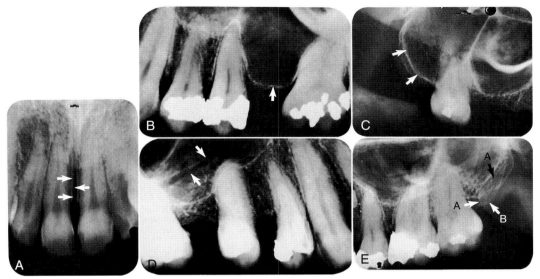

• **Fig. 14.33 II** (A) Radiograph of the medial palatine suture, the appearance of which might be interpreted as a fracture. Radiographs visualize various extensions of the maxillary sinus. (B) Alveolar extension. (C) Tuberosity extension. (D) Radiograph in which the canal for a superior alveolar artery is seen. (E) Radiograph showing typical superimposition of the coronoid process: *A*, of the mandible on the tuberosity; *B*, of the maxilla. (From McCauley HB: Anatomic characteristics important in radiodontic interpretation, *Dent Radiogr Photogr* 18:1, 1945.)

Descending Palatine and Sphenopalatine Arteries

The palatal blood supply comes from two sources but chiefly from the **descending palatine artery**, which descends from its origin from the maxillary through the greater canal. Its greater **palatine branch** enters the palate through the greater palatine foramen and runs forward with its accompanying vein and nerve in a groove at the junction of the palatine and alveolar processes. It is distributed to the bone, glands, and mucosa of the hard palate and to the bone and mucosa of the alveolar process, in which it forms anastomoses with fine branches of the superior alveolaris. Minor branches of the descending palatine artery pass to the soft palate through lesser palatine foramina in the palatine bone.

The **nasopalatine branch** of the **sphenopalatine artery** courses obliquely forward and downward on the septum and enters the palate through the incisive canal. It has a limited distribution to the incisive papilla and adjacent palate and forms an anastomosis with the greater palatine.

Nerve Supply to the Jaws and Teeth

The sensory nerve supply to the jaws and teeth is derived from the maxillary and mandibular branches of the **fifth cranial**, or **trigeminal nerve** (Fig. 14.36), whose ganglion, the trigeminal, is located at the apex of the petrous portion of the temporal bone. The innervation of the orofacial region includes, in addition to the trigeminal nerve (including V2 and V3), other cranial nerves (e.g., VII, XI, XII; Fig. 14.37).

Maxillary Nerve

The maxillary nerve (see Fig. 14.36) courses forward through the wall of the cavernous sinus and leaves the skull through the foramen rotundum.[5] It crosses the pterygopalatine fossa, where it gives branches to the pterygopalatine ganglion, a parasympathetic ganglion. This ganglion gives off several branches, now containing visceral motor and sensory fibers, to the mucous membrane of the mouth, nose, and pharynx.

The branches of clinical significance include a **greater palatine branch** that enters the hard palate through the greater palatine foramen and is distributed to the hard palate and palatal gingiva as far forward as the canine tooth; a **lesser palatine branch** from the ganglion that enters the soft palate through the lesser palatine foramina; and a **nasopalatine branch** of the posterior or superior lateral nasal branch of the ganglion that runs downward and forward on the nasal septum. Entering the palate through the incisive canal, it is distributed to the incisive papilla and to the palate anterior to the anterior palatine nerve.

The maxillary nerve also has a **posterior superior alveolar branch** from its pterygopalatine portion. This nerve enters the alveolar canals on the infratemporal surface of the maxilla and, forming a plexus, is distributed to the molar teeth and the supporting tissues.

The maxillary nerve enters the orbit and, as the **infraorbital nerve**, runs forward in its floor, first in the infraorbital groove and then in the infraorbital canal. It terminates at the infraorbital foramen in branches distributed to the upper face. At a variable distance after it enters the orbit, a **middle superior alveolar branch** arises from the infraorbital nerve and runs through the lateral wall of the maxillary sinus. It is distributed to the premolar teeth and surrounding tissues and joins the alveolar plexus. The middle superior alveolar nerve may be associated closely with the posterior superior alveolar nerve at its origin but often branches near the infraorbital foramen.

An anterior superior alveolar branch leaves the infraorbital nerve just inside the infraorbital foramen and is distributed through bony canals to the incisor and canine teeth. All three superior alveolar nerves join in a plexus above the process. From the plexus, **dental branches** are given off to each tooth root and **interdental**

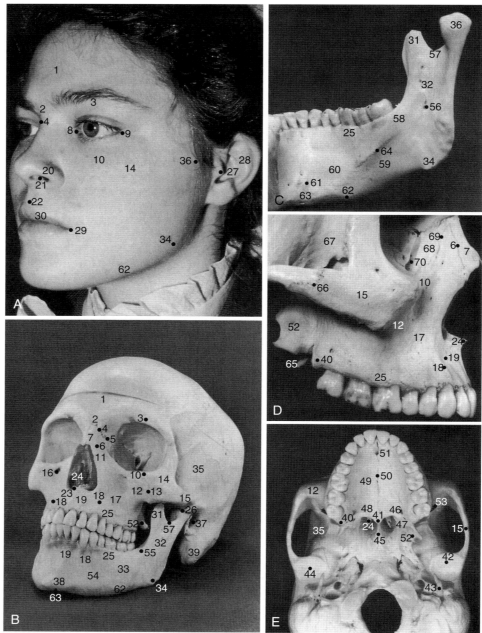

• **Fig. 14.34** Surface landmarks. Various dental structures in the patient's face can be quickly located by means of surface landmarks. Surface landmarks are identified in A. The photograph of the bony skull (B) was made from the same angle of view. Features of both are numbered and identified in the legend. The medial aspect of the mandible (C) shows anatomical details not clearly seen in the other illustrations. The maxilla and zygoma are shown in D. The bony anatomy of the hard palate and its adjoining structures is shown in E. *1,* Frontal bone (forehead); *2,* glabella; *3,* supraorbital ridge (superciliary ridge); *4,* frontonasal suture (bridge of nose); *5,* maxillofrontal suture; *6,* maxillonasal suture; *7,* nasal bone; *8,* medial canthus; *9,* lateral canthus; *10,* infraorbital ridge; *11,* frontal process of maxilla; *12,* zygomatic process of maxilla; *13,* zygomaticomaxillary suture; *14,* zygomatic bone (cheekbone); *15,* zygomatic arch; *16,* infraorbital foramen; *17,* canine fossa; *18,* canine eminence; *19,* incisive fossa; *20,* nasal ala; *21,* nares; *22,* philtrum; *23,* anterior nasal spine; *24,* inferior nasal concha; *25,* alveolar process; *26,* temporomandibular articulation; *27,* tragus of ear; *28,* auricula; *29,* labial commissure; *30,* vermilion border of lip; *31,* coronoid process of mandible; *32,* ramus of mandible; *33,* body of mandible; *34,* gonial angle of mandible; *35,* infratemporal fossa; *36,* condyle; *37,* external acoustic meatus; *38,* mental protuberance; *39,* mastoid process of temporal bone; *40,* maxillary tuberosity; *41,* posterior nasal spine; *42,* articular eminence; *43,* styloid process of temporal bone; *44,* mandibular fossa; *45,* vomer; *46,* greater palatine foramen; *47,* lesser palatine foramen; *48,* palatine bone; *49,* palatine process of maxilla; *50,* midpalatal suture; *51,* incisive foramen; *52,* lateral pterygoid plate of sphenoid bone; *53,* inferior orbital fissure; *54,* mental foramen; *55,* oblique line; *56,* mandibular foramen; *57,* mandibular notch; *58,* internal oblique ridge; *59,* submandibular fossa; *60,* sublingual fossa; *61,* genial tubercle; *62,* inferior border of mandible; *63,* symphysis; *64,* mylohyoid line; *65,* hamular process of sphenoid bone; *66,* zygomaticotemporal suture; *67,* greater wing of sphenoid bone; *68,* lacrimal bone; *69,* maxillolacrimal suture; *70,* lacrimal fossa.

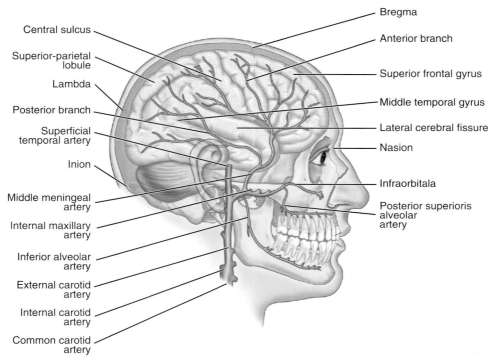

• **Fig. 14.35** Projection of maxillary artery and its branches in relation to brain, skull, and mandible, including the teeth.

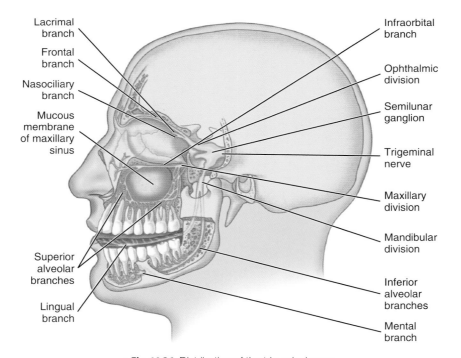

• **Fig. 14.36** Distribution of the trigeminal nerve.

branches to the bone, periodontal membrane, and gingiva, the distribution being similar to that described for the arteries.

Mandibular Nerve

The mandibular nerve (see Fig. 14.37) leaves the skull through the foramen ovale and almost immediately breaks up into its several branches. The chief branch to the lower jaw is the **inferior alveolar nerve**, which at first runs directly downward across the medial surface of the lateral pterygoid, at the lower border of which it is directed laterally and downward across the outer surface of the medial pterygoid muscle to reach the mandibular foramen. Just before entering the foramen, it releases the mylohyoid branch, which is a motor branch to the mylohyoid muscle and anterior belly of the digastric muscle.

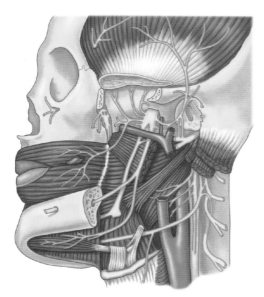

• **Fig. 14.37** Mandibular nerve. The inferior alveolar nerve branch (in the cut section of the mandible and the mandibular canal) provides innervation for the mandibular teeth. The injection of a local anesthetic into the vicinity of the lingula (see Fig. 14.17) blocks the sensory innervation of the inferior alveolar nerve and the lingual nerve ("mandibular block"), which results in a feeling of numbness of the mandibular teeth, lower lip, and side of the tongue on the side of the injection.

The inferior alveolar nerve continues forward through the mandibular canal beneath the roots of the molar teeth to the level of the mental foramen. During this part of its course, it gives off branches to the molar and premolar teeth and their supporting bone and soft tissues. The nerves to the teeth do not arise as individual branches but as two or three larger branches that form a plexus from which **inferior dental branches** enter individual tooth roots and *interdental branches* supply alveolar bone, periodontal membrane, and gingiva.

At the mental foramen, the nerve divides and a smaller incisive branch continues forward to supply the anterior teeth and bone, and a larger mental branch emerges through the foramen to supply the skin of the lower lip and chin.

Other branches of the mandibular nerve contribute in some degree to the innervation of the mandible and its investing membranes. The **buccal nerve**, although chiefly distributed to the mucosa of the cheek, has a branch that is usually distributed to a small area of the buccal gingiva in the first molar area, but in some cases, its distribution may extend from the canine to the third molar. The **lingual nerve**, as it enters the floor of the mouth, lies against the body of the mandible and has mucosal branches to a variable area of lingual mucosa and gingiva. The **mylohyoid nerve** may sometimes continue its course forward on the lower surface of the mylohyoid muscle and enter the mandible through small foramina on either side of the midline. In some individuals, it is thought to contribute to the innervation of central incisors and periodontal ligament.

Pretest Answers

1. B
2. B
3. C
4. A
5. C

References

1. Updegrave WJ: Normal radiodontic anatomy, *Dent Radiogr Photogr* 31:57, 1958.
2. MacMillan HW: The structure and function of the alveolar process, *J Am Dent Assoc* 11:1059, 1924.
3. McCauley HB: Anatomic characteristics important in radiodontic interpretation, *Dent Radiogr Photogr* 18:1, 1945.
4. Jones TS, Shepard WC: *A manual of surgical anatomy*, Philadelphia, 1945, Saunders.
5. King BG, Showers MJ: *Human anatomy and physiology*, ed 6, Philadelphia, 1969, Saunders.

Bibliography

Callander CL: *Surgical anatomy*, ed 2, Philadelphia, 1939, Saunders.
Deaver JB: *Surgical anatomy of the human body*, ed 2, Philadelphia, 1926, Blakiston.
Brash JC, Jamieson EB: Head and neck: brain. In ed 10, *Cunningham's manual of practical anatomy*, vol. 3. New York, 1940, Oxford University Press.
Morris H: *Human anatomy*, ed 10, Philadelphia, 1942, Blakiston.
Pernkopf E: Vestibulum and cavum oris, pharynx. In Femer H, editor: *Atlas of topographical and applied human anatomy: head and neck*, vol. 1. Philadelphia, 1963, Saunders. (Monsen H, translator.)
Rohen JW, Yokochi C: *Color atlas of anatomy: a photographic study of the human body*, ed 2, New York, 1988, Igaku-Shoin Medical.

approximately 1 mm.[6] Centric occlusion (or **acquired** or **habitual centric** as it is sometimes called) is a tooth-determined position, whereas centric relation is a jaw-to-jaw relation determined by the condyles in the fossae. Closure into occlusion occurs usually anterior to centric relation; however, a coincidence of centric relation contact and the intercuspal position is evident in about 10% of the population.

Rest position is a postural position of the mandible determined largely by neuromuscular activity and to a lesser degree by the viscoelastic properties of the muscles. Thus, because tonicity of muscles may be influenced by the central nervous system as a result of factors such as emotional stress and by local peripheral factors such as a sore tooth, the rest position of the mandible is not consistent. The interocclusal space with the mandible in rest position and the head in upright position is about 1 to 3 mm at the incisors but has considerable normal variance even up to 8 to 10 mm without evidence of dysfunction.

Mandibular Movements

In lateral movements (Fig. 15.14), the condyle appears to rotate with a slight lateral shift in the direction of the movement. This movement is called the **Bennett movement** and may have both immediate and progressive components. By the use of recording equipment such as a pantograph or kinesiograph, it is possible to record mandibular movements in relation to a particular plane of reference (e.g., sagittal, horizontal, or frontal planes). If a point (the incisive point) located between the incisal edges of the two mandibular central incisors is tracked during maximal lateral, protrusive, retrusive, and wide opening movements, such movements are seen to take place within a border or envelope of movements.[6] Functional and parafunctional movements occur within these borders. However, most functional movements such as those associated with mastication occur chiefly around centric. Border movements in the horizontal plane are shown in Fig. 15.14. (To view Animations 15, 16, and 17, please go to Expert Consult.)

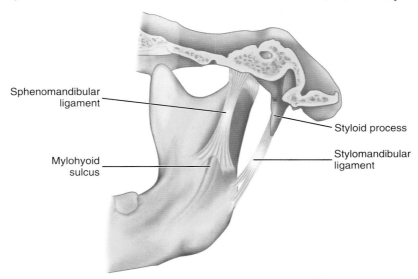

• **Fig. 15.7** Sphenomandibular and stylomandibular ligaments.

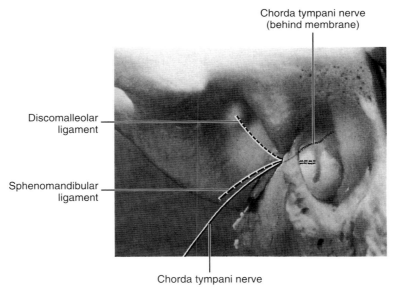

• **Fig. 15.8** Ligaments attached to the malleus. (From Ash MM, Ash CM, Ash JL, et al: Current concepts of the relationship and management of temporomandibular disorders and auditory symptoms, *J Mich Dent Assoc* 72:550–555, 1990.)

The maximum opening movement is 50 to 60 mm, depending on the age and size of the individual. An arbitrary lower limit for normal of 40 mm may be in error, inasmuch as some individuals may have no difficulty incising a large apple and have no history of TMJ muscle dysfunction. The maximum lateral movement in the absence of TMJ muscle dysfunction, including pain, is about 10 to 12 mm. The maximum protrusive movement is approximately 8 to 11 mm, again depending on the size of the subject and skull morphology. The retrusive range for adults and children is about 1 mm, although 2 to 3 mm may be observed infrequently.[7] The retrusive range, as measured from centric occlusion to centric relation, is considered a discrepancy between centric occlusion and centric relation. Border movements in the sagittal plane are shown in Fig. 15.13.

All values for border movements must be related to function—that is, a maximum lateral movement of 7 to 8 mm to the right (10 to 12 mm to the left) must be related to the occlusion and to whether translation of the left condyle occurs, because the latter may be "fixed" because of dysfunction or pain. Such values should also be related to other functions such as incising, chewing, swallowing, and speaking. However, if such values are made a part of every patient's dental record, any change can be evaluated in terms of dysfunction.

Muscles

Masticatory functions, speaking, yawning, and swallowing involve reflex contraction and relaxation of the muscles of mastication, whose activity is initiated voluntarily. It is impossible to determine clinically if a particular muscle is participating in a particular movement solely from its origin and insertion. Patterns of muscle contraction are complex and even in the same areas may have different functions.

The complex movements of the TMJ suggest that muscles of mastication exhibit differential regional action and regional differences in their histochemical profiles. Thus, to consider a "muscle" as a contracting entity is an oversimplification. In reality, each muscle is a collection of motor units with different properties located in different parts of a single muscle and exhibiting different activities. However, for obvious reasons, the action of the various muscles will be given as a contracting entity.

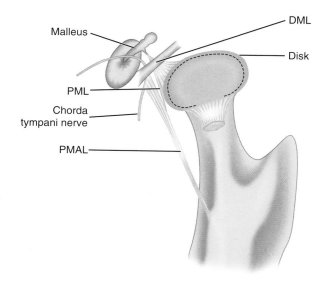

• **Fig. 15.9** Ligaments attached to the malleus. *DML,* Discomalleolar ligament fibers; *PML,* fibers from sphenomandibular ligament; *PMAL,* fibers from the discomalleolar and sphenomandibular ligament.

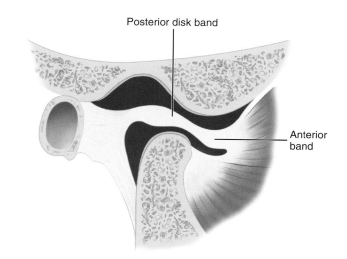

• **Fig. 15.11** Articular disk: jaw in open position.

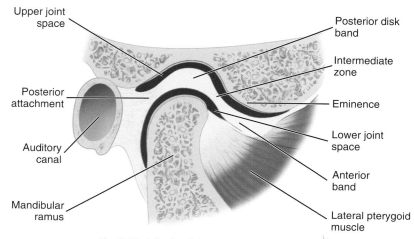

• **Fig. 15.10** Articular disk and associated structures.

The masticatory muscles concerned with mandibular movements include the lateral pterygoid, anterior digastric, masseter, medial pterygoid, and temporalis muscles. Also, the mylohyoid and geniohyoid muscles are involved in masticatory functions.

Several muscles associated with the ear, throat, and neck are of interest to the dentist, including tensors tympani and palatini, because the latter two may relate to subjective hearing disorders such as stuffiness, some forms of tinnitus, and noise.[1,8–10]

Lateral Pterygoid Muscle

The **lateral pterygoid muscle** has two origins: one head originates on the outer surface of the lateral pterygoid plate, and an upper or superior head originates on the greater sphenoid wing (Figs. 15.15, 15.16, and 15.17C). The insertion is on the anterior surface of the neck of the condyle. In addition, an insertion is evident of some fibers to the capsule of the joint and anterior aspect of the articular disk (see Fig. 15.17C).

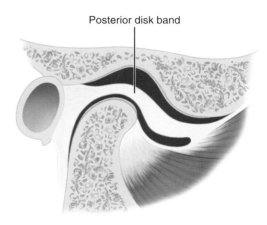

Posterior disk band

• **Fig. 15.12** Articular disk, anterior displacement: jaw in closed position.

The superior head is active during various jaw-closing movements only, whereas the inferior head is active during jaw-opening movements and protrusion only.[11] The lateral pterygoid is anatomically suited for protraction, depression, and contralateral abduction. It may also be active during other movements for joint stabilization. The superior head is active during such closing movements as chewing and clenching of the teeth and during swallowing. Presumably, the superior head positions or stabilizes the condylar head and disk against the articular eminence during mandibular closing. The inferior head assists in the translation of the condyle downward, anteriorly, and contralaterally during jaw opening. The lateral pterygoid muscle is innervated by the trigeminal nerve (V) (see Fig. 14.37).

Masseter Muscle

The **masseter muscle** extends from the zygomatic arch to the ramus and body of the mandible. The insertion of this muscle is broad, extending from the region of the second molar on the lateral surface of the mandible to the posterior lateral surface of the ramus (Figs. 15.18 and 15.19). The masseter muscle is covered partly by the platysma muscle (see Fig. 15.19) and by the risorius muscle. The platysma is activated during firm clenching in some individuals and, having some insertion in the orbicular muscle (orbicularis oris), is sometimes active in facial expression. The risorius is affected by emotion and is active in facial expression.

The superficial part of the masseter muscle is separated distinctly only from the deeper layer of the muscle at the posterior upper part of the muscle. The masseter muscle is covered partly and to a variable degree with the parotid gland tissue. The center of the lower third of the masseter muscle is about 2 to 3 cm from the anterior border of the sternocleidomastoid muscle, which contracts during clenching in some individuals. The masseter muscle is active during forceful jaw closing and may assist in protrusion of the mandible. The masseter muscle is innervated by the fifth nerve

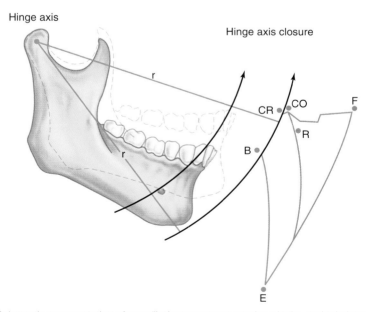

• **Fig. 15.13** Schematic representation of mandibular movement envelope in the sagittal plane. *CR*, Centric relation; *CO*, centric occlusion; *F*, maximum protrusion; *R*, rest position; *E*, maximum opening; *B* to *CR*, opening and closing on hinge axis with no change in radius *(r)*. (To view Animations 11 and 12, please go to Expert Consult.)

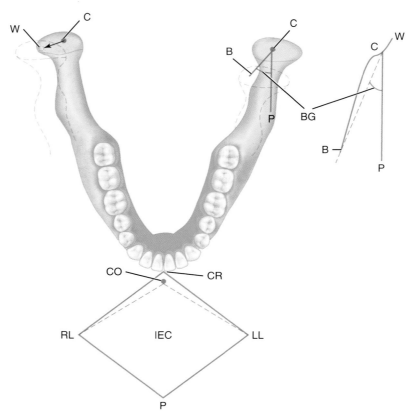

• **Fig. 15.14** Right mandibular movement with schematic representation of movement at the incisal point in the horizontal plane *(CR, LL, P, RL)* and at the condyle *(W, C, B, P)* made by a pantograph. Teeth are not in occlusion. *CR,* Centric relation; *CO,* centric occlusion; *IEC,* incisal edge contact; *LL,* left lateral; *P,* protrusive; *RL,* right lateral. On the right side, the condyle moves from *C* (centric) to right working *(W).* On the balancing side, the left condyle moves from *C* along line *B* and makes an angle *BG,* called the *Bennett angle. C* to *P,* Straight protrusive movement. (To view Animations 13 and 14, please go to Expert Consult.)

(masseter nerve). The **zygomaticomandibular muscle** (deep masseter muscle) inserts at the coronoid process and originates on the inner surface of the zygomatic arch (see Fig. 15.17B). It may be a synergist for the posterior temporalis and an antagonist for the lateral pterygoid muscle.

Medial Pterygoid Muscle

The **medial pterygoid muscle** arises from the medial surface of the lateral pterygoid plate and from the palatine bone (see Figs. 15.15 and 15.16). It inserts on the medial surface of the angle of the mandible and on the ramus up to the mandibular foramen. The principal functions of the medial pterygoid muscle are elevation and lateral positioning of the mandible. It is active during protrusion. The innervation is a branch of the mandibular division of the fifth nerve.

Temporalis Muscle

The **temporalis muscle** is fan-shaped and originates in the temporal fossa (Fig. 15.20; also see Figs. 15.16, 15.17B, and 15.18). On passing to the zygomatic arch, it forms a tendon that inserts into the anterior border and mesial surface of the coronoid process of the mandible and along the anterior border of the ascending ramus of the mandible (see Fig. 15.16). The anterior fibers extend

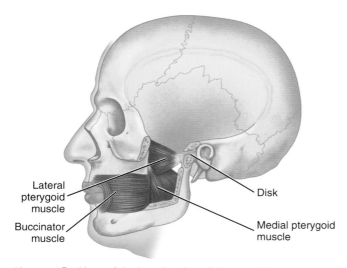

• **Fig. 15.15** Positions of the lateral and medial pterygoid muscles shown with cutaway sections of bone.

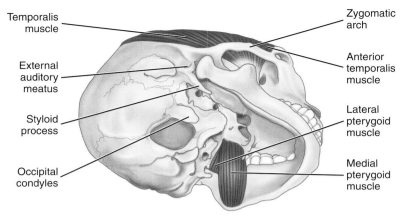

• **Fig. 15.16** View of the medial and lateral pterygoid muscles. Note the insertion of the temporalis muscle also in Fig. 15.17B.

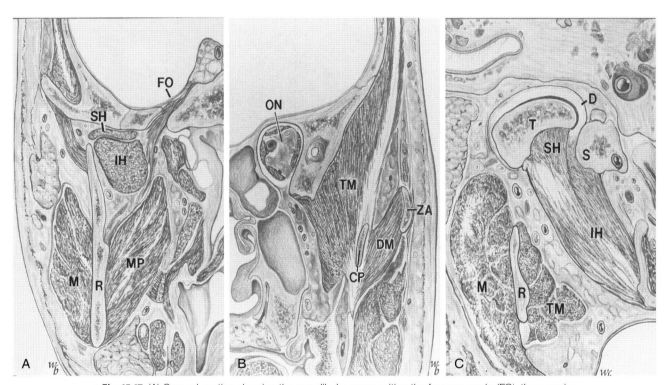

• **Fig. 15.17** (A) Coronal section showing the mandibular nerve exiting the foramen ovale *(FO)*, the superior *(SH)* and inferior *(IH)* heads of the lateral pterygoid muscle, the ascending ramus *(R)*, and the masseter *(M)* and medial pterygoid *(MP)* muscle. (B) Optic nerve *(ON)*, temporalis muscle *(TM)*, deep masseter *(DM)* or zygomaticomandibular muscle, and coronoid process *(CP)*. *ZA,* Zygomatic arch. (C) Horizontal section at the level of the temporomandibular joint, showing the condyle *(T)*, superior head of lateral pterygoid muscle *(SH)*, inferior head *(IH)*, ascending ramus *(R)*, masseter muscle *(M)*, and temporalis muscle *(TM)*. *D,* Disk; *S,* styloid. (Redrawn from Widmalm SE, Lillie JH, Ash MM: Anatomical and electromyographic studies of the lateral pterygoid muscle, *J Oral Rehabil* 14:429, 1987.)

along the anterior border of the ramus almost to the third molar. The muscle has three component parts and appears to behave as if it consisted of three distinct parts. The temporal muscle is the principal positioner of the mandible during elevation. The posterior part is active in retruding the mandible, and the anterior part is active in clenching. The anterior part may act as a synergist with the masseter in clenching, whereas the posterior part acts as an antagonist to the masseter in retruding the jaw. The temporalis muscle is innervated by temporal branches of the mandibular division of the fifth nerve.

Digastric Muscle

The attachment of the **anterior digastric muscle** is at or near the lower border of the mandible and near the midline (see Fig. 15.20). A tendon is between the anterior and posterior digastric muscles and is attached by a looplike strip of fascia to the hyoid bone. The anterior digastric muscle is covered by the platysma muscle, and beneath lie the mylohyoid and the geniohyoid muscles. All these muscles are considered to be active during various phases of jaw opening. A mylohyoid branch of the mandibular division of the fifth nerve innervates the anterior digastric muscle (see Fig. 14.37); the digastric branch of the facial nerve innervates the posterior digastric muscle.

Geniohyoid Muscle

The **geniohyoid muscle** lies superior to the mylohyoid muscle and adjacent to the midline. It arises from the mental spine on the posterior aspect of the symphysis menti of the mandible. It inserts on the anterior surface of the hyoid bone. When the mandible is fixed, the hyoid bone is drawn forward and upward; when the hyoid bone is fixed, the lower jaw is depressed. Innervation is from C1 (see Fig. 14.37).

Tensor Tympani and Palatini Muscles

The tensor tympani, tensor veli palatini, and levator veli palatini muscles (Figs. 15.21 and 15.22) may have clinical significance for

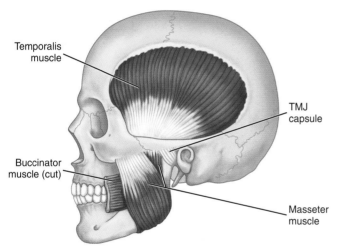

• **Fig. 15.18** Masticatory muscles shown include the temporalis and masseter muscles. The deep masseter is attached to the zygoma (see Fig. 15.17C). *TMJ,* Temporomandibular joint.

subjective auditory symptoms associated with temporomandibular and muscle disorders (TMDs).[1,8,9] The tensor tympani and tensor veli palatini muscles are innervated by the trigeminal nerve and therefore may respond to similar kinds of ascending information from joints, skin, and muscles and from descending inputs from higher centers that converge on interneurons and the trigeminal motor nucleus (Fig. 15.23). Disturbances of auditory tube opening during swallowing that may occur with TMJ and TMDs appear to be consistent with restricted function and anatomy of the tensor palatini and levator veli palatini muscles.[10] If a causal connection between subjective hearing symptoms and TMDs is to be established, additional evidence-based research is needed.

Restricted jaw opening and prevention of yawning seen in TMJ and TMDs can lead to otological symptoms such as subjective hearing loss associated with sensations of stuffiness in the ear.[1] Thus, pain in and around the joints and muscles may influence the otomandibular muscles through interneurons in the intertrigeminal area and might be responsible for a few cases of tinnitus associated with restricted jaw opening due to TMJ and muscle disorders.

Head and Neck Muscles

The muscles of the head and neck have been of interest to the dentist because of a potential relationship among the occlusion, TMJs, and pain in these muscles and/or muscle contraction headache. The possible role of the epicranius muscles in tension headache has yet to be clarified. The sternocleidomastoid muscle (see Fig. 15.20) is often affected in patients with TMJ muscle dysfunction and often co-contracts with jaw clenching. The functions of the orbicularis oris and buccinator muscles (see Fig. 15.19) appear to have a significant role for optimal function of complete dentures. The seventh (VII) nerve innervates all the muscles of facial expression.

Other muscles that are of interest to the dentist because of TMJ and muscle disorders are the scalenus, splenius, iliocostalis cervicis, and omohyoideus. However, the association between TMDs and myalgia of the muscles has not been established. A number of problems in oral motor function, such as lip posture in the aged, may be related to a generalized deterioration in performance or to a specific

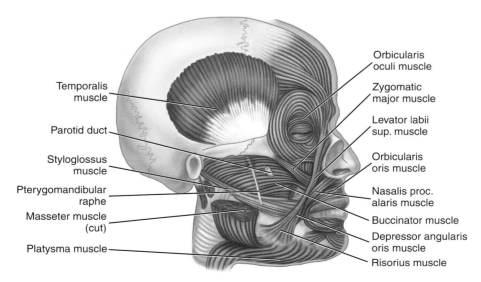

• **Fig. 15.19** Muscles of facial expression and accessory muscles of mastication. *Sup.,* Superior; *proc.,* procerus.

motor function rather than the dental state or prescription medication. Most reports on motor disorders and aging have focused on disturbances in control originating in the nervous system.

Mandibular Movements and Muscle Activity

Mandibular movement during normal function and during parafunction (e.g., bruxism) involve complex neuromuscular patterns originating in part in a pattern generator in the brainstem and modified by influences from higher centers (see Fig. 15.23), namely, the cerebral cortex and basal ganglia, and from peripheral influences (e.g., the periodontium, muscles). However, a detailed discussion of such movements is beyond the scope of this text. Rather, the discussion relates to muscle activity as seen in electromyography for jaw opening and closing, protrusion, retrusion, and lateral movements.

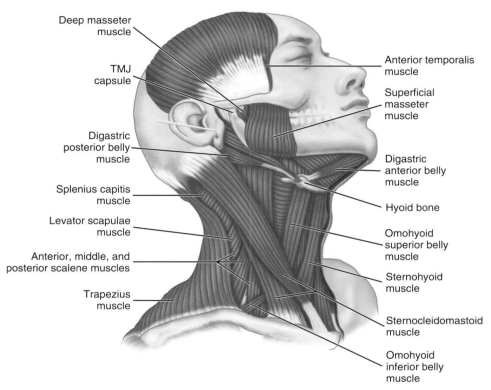

• **Fig. 15.20** Muscles of the neck. *TMJ,* Temporomandibular joint.

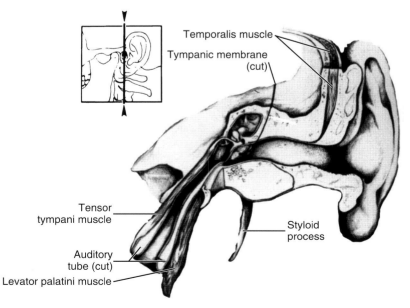

• **Fig. 15.21** Section through the ear showing inner ear structures and the tensor tympani muscle, which is active in stretching the tympanic membrane.

Mandibular Opening

The digastric, mylohyoid, and geniohyoid muscles are active during jaw opening, either slowly or maximally against resistance. No activity occurs in the temporalis and masseter muscles when the mouth is opened slowly and the jaw is opened maximally, although some activity may occur in the medial pterygoid muscle. When the jaw is opened against resistance, the temporalis muscle remains silent. During opening movements, the lateral pterygoid muscles show initial and sustained activity. In forced depression, the digastric muscle is activated almost as soon as the lateral pterygoid muscle. Generally, the activity of the anterior digastric muscle follows that of the lateral pterygoid muscle.

Mandibular Closing

While the mandible is being elevated slowly, without contact of the teeth, no activity is evident in any portion of the temporalis muscle. Elevation without contact or resistance is brought about

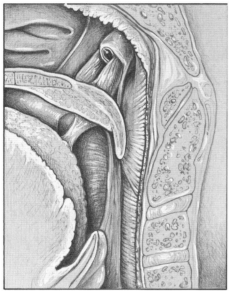

• **Fig. 15.22** Muscles of the throat. Eustachian tube and tensor palatini muscle, which is active in opening the auditory tube.

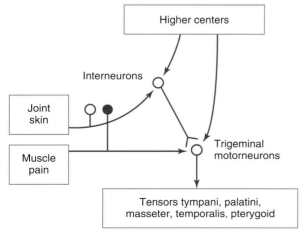

• **Fig. 15.23** Information from joints, skin, muscles, and higher centers converge on the interneurons and trigeminal motor nucleus.

by contraction of the masseter and medial pterygoid muscle. The temporalis, masseter, and medial pterygoid muscles affect elevation against resistance. The suprahyoid muscles act as an antagonist of the elevator muscles. Closure into maximal intercuspation (centric occlusion) may involve contraction of facial and neck muscles.

Retrusion

Voluntary mandibular retrusion with the mouth closed is brought about by contraction of the posterior fibers of the temporalis muscle and by the suprahyoid and infrahyoid muscles. Retraction of the mandible from protrusion and without occlusal contact is effected by the contraction of the posterior and middle fibers of the temporalis muscles. Slight activity of the suprahyoid may be the result of slight jaw opening to allow the teeth to glide over each other from centric occlusion to centric relation.

Protrusion

Protrusion of the mandible without occlusal contact results from contraction of the lateral and medial pterygoid muscles and also masseter muscles. Protraction against resistance is brought about by contraction of the lateral and medial pterygoid muscles and of the masseter and suprahyoid muscle group. Protrusion with the teeth in occlusion is achieved by contraction of the pterygoid and masseter muscles. Only slight activity occurs in the suprahyoid muscles. In combined protraction and opening, activity is evident in the medial and lateral pterygoid muscles, the masseter muscles, and sometimes the anterior fibers of the temporalis muscles.

Lateral Movements

Lateral movement of the mandible to the right side (without occlusal contact) is achieved by ipsilateral contraction of primarily the posterior fibers of the temporalis muscle. The suprahyoid muscles are active in maintaining the jaw slightly depressed and protruded. Movement to the left side without occlusal contact is brought about by the contralateral contraction of the medial pterygoid and masseter muscles. Lateral movement to the right side against resistance is achieved by the ipsilateral contraction of the temporalis muscle and by some activity in the ipsilateral masseter and medial pterygoid muscles. Movement to the left side against resistance is achieved by the contralateral contraction of the medial pterygoid and masseter muscles. Lateral movement to the right with occlusal contact is achieved by ipsilateral contraction of the temporalis muscle. Movement to the left with occlusal contact is brought about by contralateral contraction of the medial pterygoid and masseter muscles. Both lateral pterygoid muscles initiate depression of the mandible, and the contralateral muscle initiates a lateral transversion. Lateral movements of the jaw are achieved by ipsilateral contraction of the posterior and middle fibers of the temporalis muscle and by contralateral contraction of the lateral and medial pterygoid muscles and the anterior fibers of the temporalis muscle. Parts of the temporal and masseter muscles may act as antagonists or synergists during horizontal movements and minimum separation of the teeth.

Chewing

Chewing is highly complex oral motor behavior usually seen in the frontal plane in simple form (Fig. 15.24). No archetypal chewing cycle exists. The means of the dimensions of the chewing cycle are between 16 and 20 mm for vertical movements and between 3 and 5 mm for lateral movements. The duration of the cycle varies from 0.6 to 1 second depending on the type of food. The speed of masticatory movement varies within each cycle, both according to the type of food and among individuals. Speed, duration, and form of the chewing cycle vary with the type of occlusion, kind of food, and presence of dysfunction.

Occlusal contacts occur in centric occlusion in at least 80% to 90% of all chewing cycles, especially near complete trituration of the bolus. With closing and opening movements, contact gliding is seen. In the closing phase, the contact glide depends on the type of occlusion and type of food. Where tough food is the

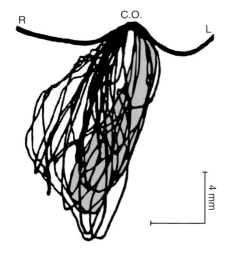

• **Fig. 15.24** Mandibular movements during the process of chewing naturally. Incisor point movement is seen in the frontal plane. *L,* Left; *CO,* centric occlusion; *R,* right. (To view Animation 13, please go to Expert Consult.)

normal diet (e.g., as with Australian aborigines) with corresponding occlusal wear, the chewing movement shows a long contact glide (2.8 ± 0.35 mm)[12] compared with the short contact glide (0.90 ± 0.36 mm) of Europeans living on a modern diet of easily triturated food.[13] The chewing force reaches a maximum in centric occlusion and lasts for 40 to 170 ms, and the peak electromyographic activity of the temporal and masseter muscles lasts for a mean of 41 ± 26 ms. Some chewing force is maintained for gliding tooth contact on the opening phase. In the intercuspal position, the jaw is stationary, or it pauses for approximately 100 ms before the next cycle begins.

Swallowing

Swallowing involves most of the tongue muscles and buccal musculature.[14] In the initial stage of swallowing, the bolus moves from the mouth to the fauces (Fig. 15.25). The bolus is then moved from the fauces to the esophagus and finally through the esophagus to the stomach. When saliva is swallowed, total participation of the suprahyoid muscles occurs, with marked activity of the digastric and mylohyoid muscles, followed by moderate activity in the geniohyoid muscles. The medial pterygoid muscle is often active; less often, the temporalis and masseter muscles are active with occlusal contact.

Oral Motor Behavior

Oral motor behavior refers to function and parafunction of the mouth and associated structures. More generally, behavior includes observable actions ranging from simple movements such as retrusion or protrusion to more complex movements such as chewing. To accomplish complex behavior, sensorimotor systems consisting of muscles and neural processes are required for the initiation, programming, and execution of motor functions.

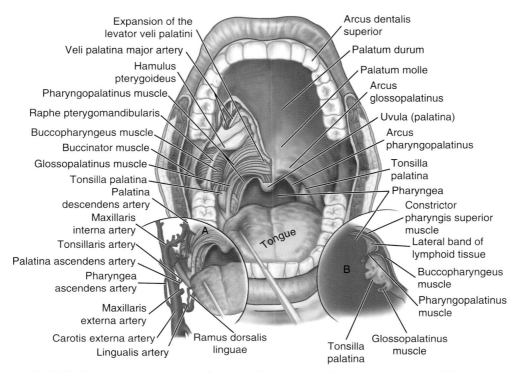

• **Fig. 15.25** Oral pharynx, with special reference to the palatine tonsil and the musculature of the palate.

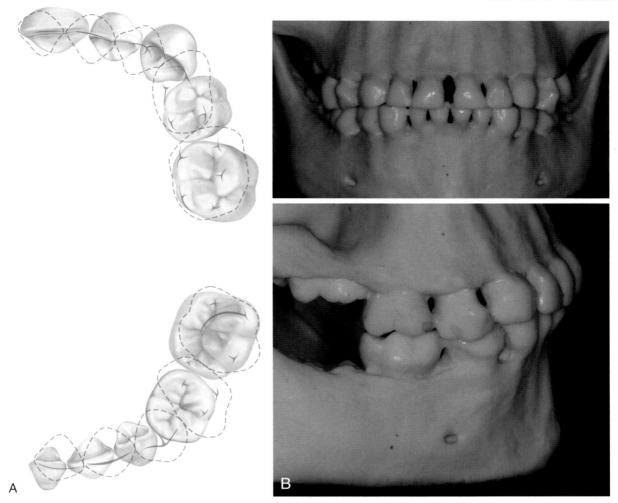

• **Fig. 16.8** Occlusal contact relations of primary dentition. (A) Contacts on maxillary teeth *(top)* and contacts on mandibular teeth *(bottom)*. (B) Model of normally developed teeth of a child 6 years of age. *Top,* Frontal view. *Bottom,* Sagittal view. (B, Model courtesy BoneClones, Osteological Reproductions.)

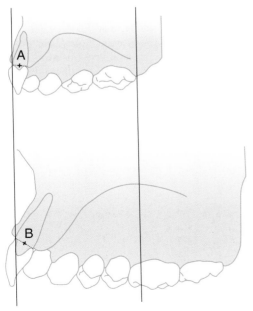

• **Fig. 16.9** Drawings of a sagittal section through the permanent and primary incisors. The labial surface at the cervical margin is oriented in the same plane. Note that the midalveolar point of the permanent incisors (B) is more lingual than the same point of the primary incisor (A) but that the incisal edge of the permanent incisor is more labial than that of the primary incisor.

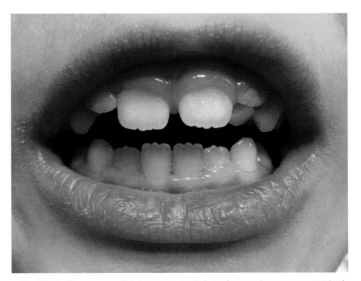

• **Fig. 16.10** Observe available space and size of emerging permanent incisors and incisal edge mamelons. Note the loss of the maxillary left primary lateral incisor as the permanent lateral incisor emerges. (Courtesy Elena Farfel, DMD, Las Vegas, NV.)

the permanent dentition. For example, the aggregate size of the posterior permanent teeth is generally smaller in the mesiodistal dimension than that of the primary teeth, and the posterior succedaneous teeth (permanent teeth) generally have a smaller total mesiodistal dimension than the primary teeth. The difference is related to the leeway space, or the amount of space gained by the difference in the mesiodistal dimensions of the premolars and the primary molars.[14,15] The average mesiodistal size of the primary dentition in that area is 47 mm, which, when compared with the succeeding aggregate tooth dimension of 42.2 mm, indicates an average gain of 4.8 mm in available space. In effect, the difference in size of the posterior succedaneous/permanent teeth and the primary teeth provides for the mesial movement of the permanent molars (Fig. 16.12). Thus, a simple comparison of tooth size of the two dentitions can indicate a need for additional space in both

dental arches as soon as the primary incisors are lost, except when sufficient interdental spacing is evident in the primary dentition.[25]

Some of the space made available by the leeway space (the difference in sizes between the premolars and primary molars) must be used for alignment of the lower incisors, because these teeth erupt with an average of 1.6 mm of crowding.[26] The mandibular molar will use the remainder of the space. This movement of the mandibular molar may correct an end-to-end molar relationship (normal for the mixed dentition) into a normal molar relationship in the permanent dentition (i.e., the mesial lingual cusp of the maxillary first molar occludes in the central fossa of the mandibular first molar, and the mesial buccal cusp of the maxillary first molar occludes between the mesial and distal buccal cusps of the mandibular first molar) (see Fig. 16.27).

Incisal Liability

If the second molars erupt before the premolars erupt fully, a significant shortening of the arch perimeter occurs, and malocclusion may be more likely to occur.[27] Because of the discrepancy in mesiodistal crown dimensions between the primary and permanent incisors, some degree of transient crowding may occur (incisal liability) at about the age of 8 to 9 years and persist until the emergence of the canines, when the space for the teeth may again be adequate.

Permanent Dentition

The sequence of eruption of the permanent dentition is more variable than that of the primary dentition and does not follow the same anteroposterior pattern. In addition, significant differences in the eruption sequences between the maxillary arch and the mandibular arch do not appear in the eruption of the primary dentition (Table 16.3).

The most common sequences of eruption in the maxilla are 6-1-2-4-3-5-7-8 and 6-1-2-4-5-3-7-8. The most common sequences for the mandibular arch are (6-1)-2-3-4-5-7-8 and (6-1)-2-4-3-5-7-8.[28] These are also the most favorable sequences for the prevention of malocclusion (Fig. 16.13). As noted earlier, should the second molars erupt before the premolars are fully erupted, significant shortening of the arch perimeter resulting in malocclusion is likely to occur, even if the alveolar bone arch dimensions are adequate for the size of the permanent dentition.[27]

The eruption of permanent teeth also follows the tendency for the mandibular tooth of one type to erupt before the maxillary tooth erupts. This tendency is reversed in the premolar eruption sequence. This is the result of the difference in eruption timing of the canines in the two arches. In the mandibular arch, the canine erupts before the premolar, whereas in the maxillary arch the canine generally erupts after the premolar.

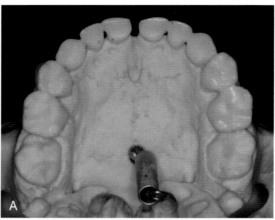
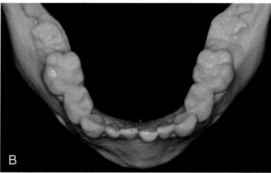

• **Fig. 16.11** Early mixed dentition in a child with a full complement of primary teeth and first permanent molars. (A) Maxilla. (B) Mandible. (Model courtesy BoneClones, Osteological Reproductions.)

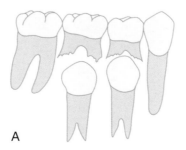
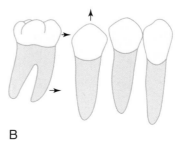

• **Fig. 16.12** Leeway space. Difference in mesiodistal dimensions between primary teeth (A) and permanent teeth (B). Arrows indicate the mesial movement of the permanent molars after loss of primary molars and eruption of the second permanent premolar.

TABLE 16.3	Chronology of Permanent Teeth		
	Tooth		**Eruption (Years)**
Upper	Cl	8, 9	7–8
	LI	7, 10	8–9
	C	6, 11	11–12
	P1	5, 12	10–11
	P2	4, 13	10–12
	m1	3, 14	9–10
	m2	2, 15	12–13
	m3	1, 16	17–21

Maxillary Teeth

Right	1	2	3	4	5	6	7	8	9	10	11	12	13	14	15	16	Left
	32	31	30	29	28	27	26	25	24	23	22	21	20	19	18	17	

Mandibular Teeth

Lower	Cl	24, 25	6–7
	LI	23, 26	7–8
	C	22, 27	9–10
	P1	21, 28	10–12
	P2	20, 29	11–12
	m1	19, 30	6–7
	m2	18, 31	11–13
	m3	17, 32	17–21

aUniversal 1 numbering system for the permanent dentition (see Chapter 1). See Tables 2.3 and 2.4 for a detailed presentation of the data.

C, Canine; *Cl,* Central incisor; *LI,* lateral incisor; *m1,* first molar; *m2,* second molar; *m3,* third molar.

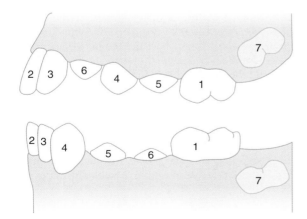

• **Fig. 16.13** Favorable emergence sequence (numerical) of permanent teeth.

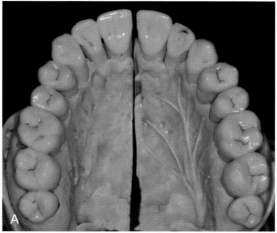

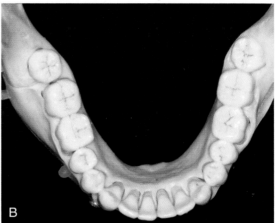

• **Fig. 16.14** The curvature of the maxillary (A) and mandibular (B) arches as seen from the occlusal (horizontal) plane tends to be maintained even though the tipped third molars alter the curvature (curve of Spee) of the arches as seen from the sagittal plane. (Model courtesy Marcus Sommer SOMSO Modelle GmbH.)

The timing of eruption of the permanent dentition is not critical as long as the eruption times are not too far from the normal values. The sequence of eruption varies somewhat, with the dentition in girls erupting an average of 5 months earlier than that in boys. However, gender differences are less significant than the tendency exhibited by the individual in the eruption times of previously erupted teeth. If any tooth has erupted early or late, succeeding teeth will also be early or late in their eruption.

Dental Arch Form

The teeth are positioned on the maxilla and mandible in such a way as to produce a curved arch when viewed from the occlusal surface (Fig. 16.14). This arch form is in large part determined by the shape of the underlying basal bone.

Malpositioning of individual teeth does not alter the arch form. When multiple teeth are misplaced, however, then irregularities or asymmetries may develop in arch form. A tapered arch form generally occurs in the maxillary arch and is quite often the result of a pathological narrowing of the anterior maxilla. Less frequently, a severe thumb-sucking habit may result in arch narrowing of the anterior maxilla (Fig. 16.15).

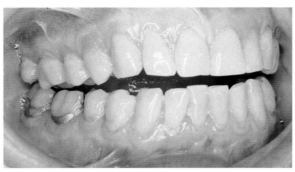

• **Fig. 16.15** Anterior open bite. (From Dawson PE: *Functional occlusion: from TMJ to smile design*, St Louis, 2007, Mosby.)

The basic pattern of tooth position is the arch. On the basis of qualitative observations, anthropologists have described the general shape of the palatal arch as being paraboloid, U-shaped, ellipsoid, rotund, and horseshoe-shaped.[29,30] An arch has long been known architecturally (as the word *architecture* itself implies) as a strong, stable arrangement with forces being transmitted normal to the apex of a catenary curve.[31,32] The shape of the arch form of the facial surfaces of the teeth was thought by Currier[33] to be a segment of an ellipse. In the past, interest in arch form was directed toward finding an "ideal" or basic mean arch form pattern that functionally interrelates alveolar bone and teeth and could have clinical application. However, any ideal arch pattern tends to ignore variance, a clinical reality which suggests that adaptation mechanisms are more important for occlusal stability than any ideal template.

Changes in arch form, within anatomical limits, have no significant effect on occlusion unless the change is in only one of the two dental arches. Discrepancies in arch form between the maxillary and mandibular arches generally result in poor occlusal relationships. Arch form distortion in only one arch can be advantageous when the basal bone structure is incorrectly positioned, as in severe mandibular retrognathism or prognathism. In such cases, the arch form distortion in one arch allows a better occlusion on the posterior aspect than is otherwise possible.

Overlap of the Teeth

The arch form of the maxilla tends to be larger than that of the mandible. As a result, the maxillary teeth "overhang" the mandibular teeth when the teeth are in centric occlusion (the position of maximal intercuspation). The lateral or anteroposterior aspect of this overhang is called **overjet,** a term that can be made more specific, as indicated in Fig. 16.16. This relationship of the arches and teeth has functional significance, including the possibility of increased duration of occlusal contacts in protrusive and lateral movements in incising and mastication.

The significance of vertical and horizontal overlap has to be related to mastication, jaw movements, speech, type of diet, and esthetics. Excessive vertical overlap of the anterior teeth may result in tissue impingement and is referred to as an **impinging overbite** (Fig. 16.17). Correction is not simply a matter of trying to increase vertical dimension by restorations on posterior teeth. Orthodontics is generally required, and sometimes orthognathic surgery is recommended.

Gingivitis and periodontitis may occur from continued impinging overbite. The degree of vertical and horizontal overlap should be sufficient to allow jaw movement in function without interference. There should be sufficient vertical overlap (with the cuspid providing the primary guidance) to enable the disocclusion of the posterior teeth. Such movement in masticatory function is controlled

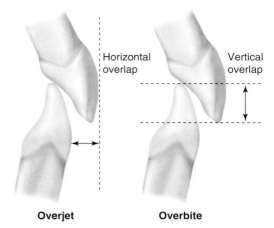

Horizontal overlap / Vertical overlap

Overjet   Overbite

• **Fig. 16.16** The terms *overjet* and *overbite* are commonly used to describe horizontal and vertical overlap of teeth.

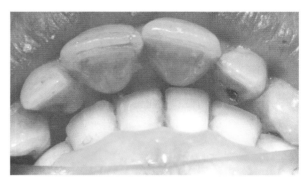

• **Fig. 16.17** Impinging overbite. (From Dawson PE: *Functional occlusion: from TMJ to smile design*, St Louis, 2007, Mosby.)

by neuromuscular mechanisms developed out of past learning in relation to physical contact of the teeth. When protective reflexes are bypassed in parafunction, trauma from occlusion involving the teeth, supporting structures, and TMJs may occur. However, aside from cheek biting as a result of insufficient horizontal overlap of the molars and trauma to the gingiva from an impinging overbite, no convincing evidence shows that a certain degree of overbite or overjet is optimal for effective mastication or stability of the occlusion. Providing the correct vertical and/or horizontal overlap requires appropriate knowledge of dental morphology, esthetics, phonetics, restorative dentistry, function, and orthodontics.

The overlapping of the maxillary teeth over the mandibular teeth has a protective feature: during opening and closing movements of the jaws, the cheeks, lips, and tongue are less likely to be caught. Because the facial occlusal margins of the maxillary teeth extend beyond the facial occlusal margins of the mandibular teeth and the linguo-occlusal margins of the mandibular teeth extend lingually in relation to the linguo-occlusal margins of the maxillary teeth, the soft tissues are displaced during the act of closure until the teeth have had an opportunity to come together in occlusal contact. Cheek biting is commonly associated with dental restorations of second permanent molars that have been made with an end-to-end occlusal relationship (i.e., without overjet).

Curvatures of Occlusal Planes

The occlusal surfaces of the dental arches do not generally conform to a flat plane (e.g., the mandibular arch has one or more curved planes conforming to the arrangement of the teeth in the dental

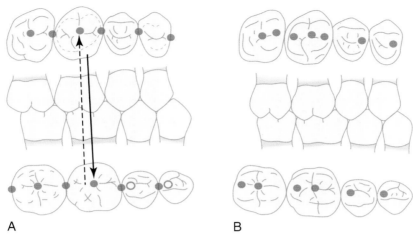

• **Fig. 16.27** Example of idealized cusp-fossa relationship. (A) Mesiolingual cusp of maxillary first molar occludes in the central fossa of the mandibular first molar. Distal buccal cusp of mandibular first molar occludes in the central fossa of the maxillary first molar. (B) Concept of occlusion in which all supporting cusps occlude in fossae.

molar (Figs. 16.27 and 16.28, first molar views).[6–8] The clinical application of the occlusal scheme of contacts shown in Fig. 16.27 is based on the concept of obtaining occlusal stability (e.g., in the intercuspal position, as in clenching, occlusal forces should be directed along the long axes of the teeth). An idealized schematic representation of all centric stops is shown in Fig. 16.29.

Lingual views of the occlusal relations with the teeth in centric occlusion (Fig. 16.30) show the intercuspation of lingual cusps and how far the maxillary teeth occlude laterally to the lingual cusps of the mandibular arch (Fig. 16.31).

Figures and legends featuring landmarks on teeth are repeated here for use as a ready reference for identifying occlusal contacts (Figs. 16.32 through 16.35).

Cusp, Fossa, and Marginal Ridge Relations

The contact relationship of the supporting cusps of the molars and premolars and fossae of the opposing teeth is shown in Fig. 16.36. The simulated relationship does not reflect all the variance that may occur in these relationships. The lingual cusps of the maxillary premolars do not necessarily make contact in the fossa of the mandibular but occlude with the marginal ridges of the premolars or premolars and first molars, as indicated in Figs. 16.36A and 16.37.

Concept of 138 Points of Occlusal Contact

One scheme of occlusal contacts presented by Hellman[8] included 138 points of possible occlusal contacts for 32 teeth. Later, with some modifications for application to complete occlusal restoration, most of the same contacts were made a part of the concept of occlusion in which supporting cusps and opposing stops (in centric relation) are tripoded and, with lateral/protrusive movements, immediate disocclusion of the posterior teeth takes place with canine (cuspid) guidance.

The list of occlusal contacts (total, 138) follows:
1. Lingual surfaces of maxillary incisors and canines, 6
2. Labial surface of mandibular incisors and canines, 6
3. Triangular ridges of maxillary buccal cusps of premolars and molars, 16

4. Triangular ridges of lingual cusps of mandibular premolars and molars, 16
5. Buccal embrasure of mandibular premolars and molars, 8
6. Lingual embrasures of maxillary premolars and molars (including the canine and first premolar embrasure accommodating the mandibular premolar), 10
7. Lingual cusp points of maxillary premolars and molars, 16
8. Buccal cusp points of mandibular premolars and molars, 16
9. Distal fossae of premolars, 8
10. Central fossae of the molars, 12
11. Mesial fossae of the mandibular molars, 6
12. Distal fossae of the maxillary molars, 6
13. Lingual grooves of the maxillary molars, 6
14. Buccal grooves of the mandibular molars, 6[a]

Therefore, if a complete description without the omission of any detail of ideal occlusion is desired, close scrutiny of a good skull or casts showing 32 teeth would make it possible to compile a list of all ridge–sulcus combinations, all cusp–embrasure combinations, and so on. Usually, if the combinations of points mentioned in the previous discussions can be established, some details, such as the approximate location of hard contact in occlusion, are automatic. Friel's concept of occlusal contacts in an "ideal" occlusion is illustrated in Fig. 16.37.[43] Compare with the contacts in Fig. 16.29.

Concepts of ideal occlusion are used primarily in orthodontics and restorative dentistry. Application of the goal of a total of 138 points for orthodontics and complete oral restorative rehabilitation has not been shown to be practical or necessary for occlusal stability or function. That is not to say that such concepts for ideal occlusal contacts have no value. Reasonable application of an idealized cusp-fossa relationship, as indicated in Figs. 16.27 and 16.37, are applicable to clinical dentistry. A complete set of the contacts in Fig. 16.37 is not a common feature of the natural dentition.

---

[a]Hellman did not list the distobuccal groove of the mandibular first molar, possibly because it is normally out of occlusal contact.

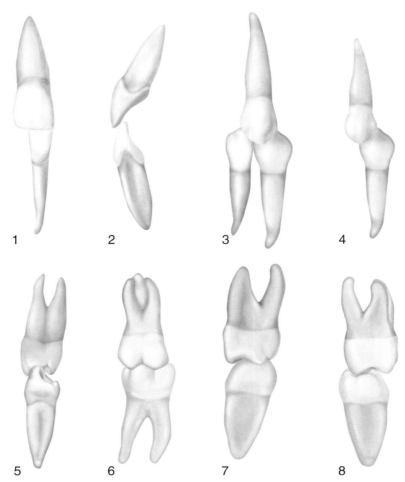

1   2   3   4

5   6   7   8

• **Fig. 16.28** Normal intercuspation of maxillary and mandibular teeth. *1*, Central incisors (labial aspect). *2*, Central incisors (mesial aspect). *3*, Maxillary canine in contact with mandibular canine and first premolar (facial aspect). *4*, Maxillary first premolar and mandibular first premolar (buccal aspect). *5*, Maxillary first premolar and mandibular first premolar (mesial aspect). *6*, First molars (buccal aspect). *7*, First molars (mesial aspect). *8*, First molars (distal aspect).

Occlusal Contact Relations and Intercuspal Relations of the Teeth

The paths made by the supporting cusps of the maxillary and mandibular first molars in lateral and protrusive mandibular movements serve to illustrate the relationship of these cusps to the morphological features of these teeth (Fig. 16.38).

Movements Away from Centric/Eccentric Movements

Occlusal contact relations away from the intercuspal position (centric occlusion) involve all possible movements of the mandible within the envelope of border movements (shown in Figs. 15.13 and 15.14). These movements are generally referred to as **lateral, lateral protrusive, protrusive, and retrusive movements.** Lateral and lateral protrusive movements may be either to the right or to the left. Designations of lateral movement often do not include lateral protrusive movements, so that basic movements are reduced to right and left lateral movement, protrusive movement, and retrusive movement. (To view Animations 18–21, please go to Expert Consult.)

Lateral Movements

During the right lateral movement, the mandible is depressed, the dental arches are separated, and the jaw moves to the right and brings the teeth together at points to the right of the intercuspal position (centric occlusion) in right working (Fig. 16.39A). On the left side, called the **nonworking** side (or, for complete dentures, the balancing side), the teeth may or may not make contact (Fig. 16.39C). Condylar movement on the working side is termed a *laterotrusive* movement in the horizontal plane. The nonworking-side condylar movement is a *mediotrusive* movement.[44]

Tooth Guidance

Concepts of occlusion often describe idealized contact relations in lateral movements as shown in Fig. 16.40. However, in the natural dentition, a variety of contact relations may be found, including group function, cuspid disocclusion only, or some combination of canine, premolar, and molar contacts in lateral movements. **Group function** refers to multiple contacts in lateral or eccentric mandibular movements (Fig. 16.41A) rather than simply **canine** (cuspid) **guidance** (see Fig. 16.41B). **Incisal guidance** refers to

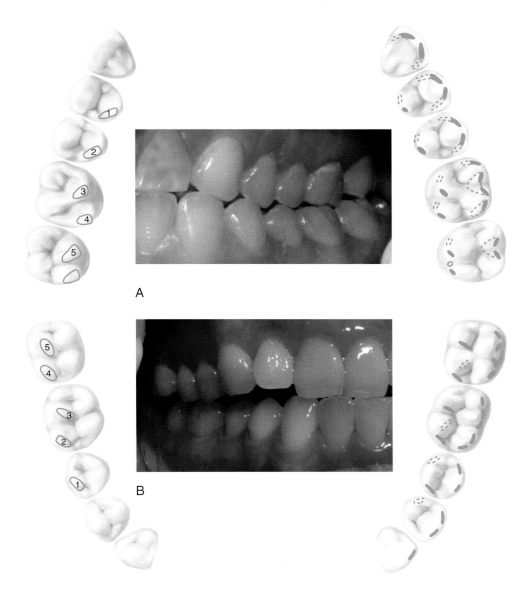

• **Fig. 16.40** (A) Patient's left side showing left working side contacts (group function) and schematic of working-side occlusal contacts and guiding inclines in left lateral movement. (B) Patient's right side showing nonworking-side occlusal contacts and guiding inclines. Nonworking contacts are not necessary except in complete dentures.

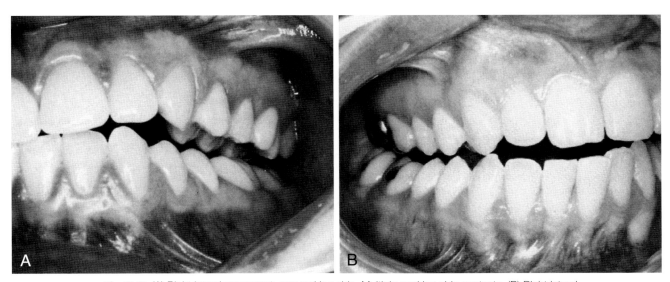

• **Fig. 16.41** (A) Right lateral movement: nonworking side. Multiple working side contacts. (B) Right lateral movement: canine (cuspid) guidance on working side.

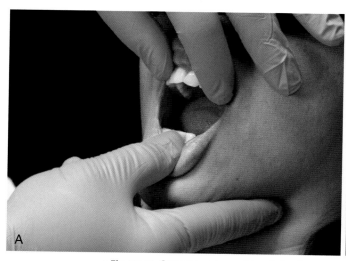
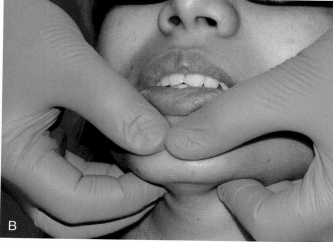

• **Fig. 16.42** Guidance into centric relation by clinician. (A) One-handed guidance. (B) Two-handed guidance.

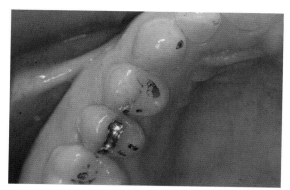

• **Fig. 16.43** Typical CRC prematurity located on maxillary first premolar. Intercuspal position marked in blue articulation paper and CRC prematurity marked in red.

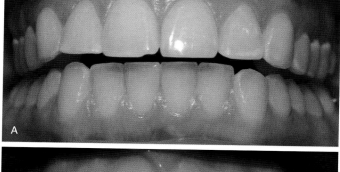
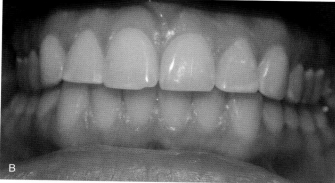

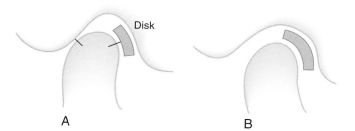

• **Fig. 16.44** (A) Incorrect assumption about the normal position of the disk-condyle assembly. (B) Correct position of the assembly in centric relation.

• **Fig. 16.45** Differences in jaw position between centric relation and the intercuspal position/centric occlusion position. (A) Centric relation. (B) Intercuspal position/centric occlusion.

Occlusal Cycle in the Molar Areas During Right or Left Lateral Occlusal Relations

In lateral movements during mastication, the mandible drops downward and to the right or left of centric occlusion. As it continues the cycle of movement and returns toward centric occlusion, the bucco-occlusal portions of mandibular molars come into contact with the occlusal portions of the maxillary molars lingual to the summits of buccal cusps and in contact with the triangular ridges of the slopes on each side of them, continuing the sliding contact until centric occlusion is accomplished (Fig. 16.49; see also Fig. 16.39).

From these first contacts, the mandibular molars slide into centric occlusion with maxillary molars and then come to a momentary rest. The movement continues with occlusal surfaces in sliding contact until the linguo-occlusal slopes of the buccal portions of the mandibular molars pass the final points of contact with the linguo-occlusal slopes of the lingual portions of the maxillary molars. When the molars lose contact, the mandible drops away in a circular movement to begin another cycle of lateral jaw movement (see Fig. 16.49).

The actual distance traveled by mandibular molars in contact across the occlusal surfaces of maxillary molars, from first contacts

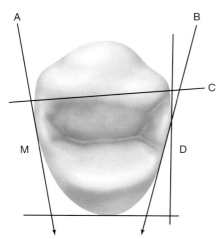

• **Fig. 16.46** Occlusion of right maxillary first premolar with its distal *(D)* and lingual surfaces surveyed by a right angle distolingually (see Fig. 9.15). *A,* Line following the angulation of the mesial surface *(M),* which is somewhat parallel with the vertical line of the right angle distally. This formation allows a proper contact relationship with the distal proximal surface of the maxillary canine; simultaneously, it cooperates with the canine in keeping the lingual embrasure design within normal limitations. *B,* Line demonstrating a more extreme angulation of the distal portion of the first premolar. This form allows cusp and ridge to bypass mandibular teeth over the distal marginal ridge surface of the maxillary tooth with normal jaw movements during lateral occlusal relations. *C,* Line aligned with mesiobuccal and distobuccal line angles, demonstrating the adaptation of the form of the buccal surface of the crown to the dental arch form without changing the functional position of the crown and root.

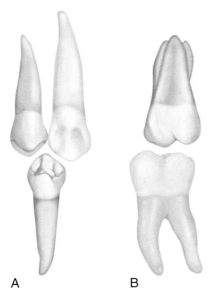

• **Fig. 16.47** Lingual aspect. Interrelationship of cusp, ridges, and embrasures. (A) Mandibular first premolar relation to maxillary canine and the first premolar approaching occlusal contact. (B) Mandibular first molar relation to the maxillary first molar on the verge of occlusal contact.

to final contacts at separation, is very short. When measured at the incisors, it is only 2.8 mm in Australian aborigines and only half or less of this in Europeans.[47] The lower molars, which are the moving antagonists, are taken out of contact before the first contact location on their buccal cusps reaches the final points of contact on the maxillary molars (compare *A* and *C* in Fig. 16.39).

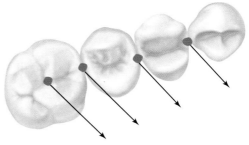

• **Fig. 16.48** Arrows indicate path of left lateral movement of mandibular teeth over the maxillary teeth on nonworking side. Note the relationship of paths to morphological features of the teeth and embrasures.

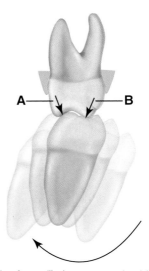

• **Fig. 16.49** Schematic of mandibular movements at the mesial aspect of the first molars. Heavy outline represents the molar in intercuspal position/centric occlusion. Shadow outlines represent mandibular molar in various relations in the movement cycle during mastication. The short arrows (A and B) at right angles to the occlusal surface of the maxillary molar measure the extent of movement between them over the occlusal surface from first contact of the mandibular molar to last contact in the cycle before starting the next cycle.

Biomechanics of Chewing Function

During the masticatory process, the individual generally chews on one side only at any one chewing stroke. Material is shifted from one side to the other when convenient; the shifting is generally confined to the molar and premolar regions, which do most of the work. Occasionally, for specific reasons the shift of mastication may be directed anteriorly. Nevertheless, the major portion of the work of mastication is done by the posterior teeth of the right or left side. The posterior teeth are aided in various ways by the canines, but the latter do not possess the broad occlusal surfaces required for chewing efficiency overall.

The tongue, lips, and cheeks manipulate the food so that it is thrown between the teeth continuously during the mandibular movements, which bring the teeth together in their various relations. In other words, the major portion of the work is accomplished in the premolar and molar regions while the mandible is making right lateral and left lateral movements, bringing the teeth into right lateral and left lateral occlusal relation and terminating the strokes in or near the intercuspal position and centric occlusion.

Protrusive Occlusal Relations

The anterior teeth in their protrusive occlusal relations negotiate the process of biting or shearing food material.

Although the mandible may be lowered considerably in producing a wide opening of the mouth, the occlusion of the anterior teeth is not concerned with any arrangement very far removed from centric relation.

When the jaw is opened and moved directly forward to the normal protrusive relation, the mandibular arch bears a forward, or anterior, relation of only 1 or 2 mm in most cases to its centric relation with the maxillary arch.

The protrusive occlusal relation places the labioincisal areas of the incisal ridges of the mandibular incisors in contact with the linguoincisal areas of the incisal portions of the maxillary incisors. The mesiolabial portion of the mesial cusp ridge of the mandibular canine should be in contact with the maxillary lateral incisors distolinguoincisally.

From the protrusive occlusal relation, the teeth glide over each other in a retrusive movement of the mandible, a movement that terminates in centric occlusion. During this final shearing action, the incisal ridges of the lower incisors are in continuous contact with the linguoincisal third portions of the maxillary incisors, from the position of protrusive occlusal relation to the return to centric occlusal relation.

The maxillary canines may assist by having their distal cusp ridges in contact with the mesial cusp of the mandibular first premolar. They cooperate with the incisors most of the time in one way or another. A slight movement to the right or left during protrusion will bring the canines together in a "biting" manner. In addition, at the end of the incisive cycle, the contact of the canines with each other in centric occlusion lends final effectiveness to the process.

Neurobehavioral Aspects of Occlusion

Up to this point, the emphasis has been on the structural, anatomical alignment of the teeth. Chapter 15 mentions briefly some of the aspects of mandibular positions and movements and muscle function. In addition, although it would be impossible to do justice to the topic of the neuroscience of occlusion in a brief review, it is imperative to call attention to the meaning of *occlusion* in its broadest sense.

Recent ideas concerning the diagnosis and treatment of disturbances such as chronic orofacial pain, temporomandibular disorders, craniomandibular disorders, and bruxism and the diagnosis and treatment of malocclusion involving orthognathic surgery require a greater knowledge of the neurobehavioral aspects of oral motor behavior than ever before in the practice of dentistry.

The neurobehavioral aspects of occlusion relate to function and parafunction of the stomatognathic system. Function includes a variety of actions or human behavior such as chewing, sucking, swallowing, speech, and respiration. *Parafunction* refers to action such as bruxism (e.g., clenching and grinding of the teeth). All these functions require highly developed sensorimotor mechanisms. The coordination of occlusal contacts, jaw motion, and tongue movement during mastication requires an intricate control system involving a number of guiding influences from the teeth and their supporting structures, TMJs, masticatory muscles, and higher centers in the central nervous system. Frequent contact of the teeth during mastication without biting the tongue; closure of the jaw to facilitate swallowing (occurring about 600 times a day);

remarkable tactile sensitivity in which threshold values for detecting foreign bodies between the teeth may be as little as 8 μm; and the presence of protective reflexes suggest the need for intricate mechanisms of control of jaw position and occlusal forces.

The presence of several classes of teeth, powerful musculature, and a most delicate positional control system indicates that it is important to understand the strategy underlying such sensitive control mechanisms. Although the ease with which these mechanisms may be disturbed at the periphery (i.e., teeth, joints, periodontium, peripheral neural system) and centrally (brainstem and higher centers) is not well understood, the adaptive capacity of the stomatognathic system appears to be considerable. On an individual clinical basis, however, the responses of a patient to occlusal therapy may be reflected in oral behavior outside the range of normal. Inasmuch as function and parafunction share similar anatomical, physiological, and psychological substrates, it is necessary to review briefly the neurobehavioral correlates of the activities of the stomatognathic system.

Occlusal Stability

The stability of the occlusion and the maintenance of tooth position are dependent on all the forces that act on the teeth. Occlusal forces, eruptive forces, lip and cheek pressure, periodontal support, and tongue pressure are all involved in maintaining the position of the teeth. As long as all these forces are balanced, the teeth and the occlusion will remain stable. Should one or more of the influences change in magnitude, duration, or frequency, stability is lost and the teeth will shift, disrupting a previously stable occlusion. The loss of teeth, tooth structure, or occlusal supporting cusps or a decrease in their support from periodontal disease or trauma is a factor in maintaining occlusal stability.

Occlusal stability refers to the tendency of the teeth, jaws, joints, and muscles to remain in an optimal functional state. The mechanisms involved include mesial migration of teeth, eruption of teeth to compensate for occlusal wear or intrusion by occlusal forces, remodeling of bone, protective reflexes and control of occlusal forces, reparative processes, and a number of others even less understood than those just listed. Although the strategy for stability related to the functional level required for survival appears obvious, orchestration of such diverse mechanisms can be couched only in terms such as **homeostasis.** The influence on occlusal stability of such factors as disease, aging, and dysfunction has yet to be clarified.

From a clinical standpoint, several concepts of occlusal stability are used as goals for occlusal therapy, including maintenance of a stable jaw relation in centric occlusion and centric relation; direction of occlusal forces along the long axis of a tooth; maintenance of centric stops, supporting cusps, and contact vertical dimension; replacement of lost teeth; and control of tooth mobility. Discussion of these aspects of occlusal stability is more appropriately found in books on occlusion.

Mesial migration is a term used to describe the migration of teeth in a mesial direction. The cause of this phenomenon has not been fully clarified, although a number of ideas have been advanced. There seems to be little doubt that mesial drift does occur, but no general agreement is evident on how much movement occurs, which teeth move, and how the movement is achieved. Suggested causes include traction of the transseptal fiber system,[48] forces of mastication,[49,50] and tongue pressure.[51] The strategy behind the mesial migration appears to be related to closure of proximal tooth contacts. Although occlusal forces may

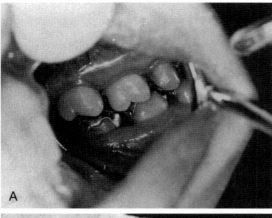

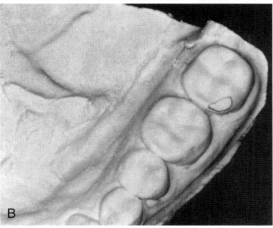

• **Fig. 16.50** (A) Opening of contact between mandibular molars due to a protrusive interference on the second molar (mirror view of left side). (B) Outline of excessive restored mesial buccal cusp ridge, which involved protrusive bruxing by the patient.

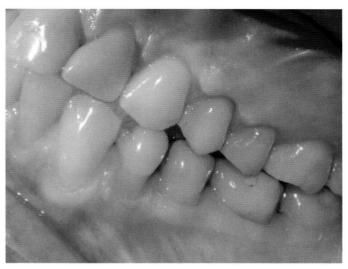

• **Fig. 16.51** Occlusal instability cannot be determined simply on the basis of occlusal contact relations and spacing of the teeth. A changing occlusion that restabilizes suggests adaptation.

be considered as a passive mechanism and traction of transseptal fibers as an active one, it is difficult to determine in what way occlusal stability is influenced. The contact relations of the teeth may promote occlusal stability, but if incorrect relations are present, opening of proximal contacts can occur (Fig. 16.50).

A tendency exists to assume that a particular arrangement of teeth is unstable (Fig. 16.51); however, such an occlusal relationship may have become stabilized, at least at a particular point in time. Whether an occlusion is fully stable can be determined only by periodic evaluation of that occlusion. Many factors (caries, periodontal disease, occlusal trauma, bruxism) may upset the delicate balance of an already marginally stable occlusion.

An ideal occlusion may be defined as one that has no structural, functional, or neurobehavioral characteristics that tend to interfere with occlusal stability. A response to bruxism may be loss of tooth structure, increased tooth mobility, root resorption (Fig. 16.52), or decreased tooth mobility and increased density and thickness of the supporting tissues.

Guidance of Occlusion

Guidance of occlusion is usually discussed only in terms of tooth contact or anatomical or physical guidance, and more specifically in relation to canine and incisal guidance. Less specific is the term **anterior guidance,** which may refer to tooth guidance for all or any of the anterior teeth or to guidance involving the

neuromuscular system. Yet another type of guidance is condylar (disk-condylar complex) guidance, which, like incisal guidance, may refer to so-called mechanical equivalents of guidance on an articulator. Again, as with anterior guidance, the neuromuscular aspects of condylar guidance are not well understood. The paths of the condyles in the mandibular fossae are not well represented in the mechanical equivalents of an articulator, especially in less than a "fully adjustable" articulator; and neuromuscular mechanisms are not represented at all.

It is of particular importance to the clinician to make certain that physical guidance of a restoration (or of the natural teeth in the treatment of dysfunction or malocclusion) is in harmony with the neuromuscular system and neurobehavioral attributes of the patient. Although some degree of compatibility may be assured through evaluation of occlusal relations and determination that smooth gliding movements are present in various excursions, the acceptance and adaptability of the neuromuscular system may not be apparent until an unfavorable response occurs (Fig. 16.53).

Adaptation

In an ideal occlusion, there should be no need for adaptation, but the criteria for it can be guidelines only, because their implementation may reflect clinical skill beyond the ordinary. Even minor occlusal discrepancies in a few individuals may result in acute orofacial pain and/or TMJ and muscle symptoms. It is not uncommon to have some kind of response (structural function and/or psychological) after the restoration of a maxillary central incisor if an occlusal interference to complete closure in centric occlusion has been placed by mistake in the restoration (Fig. 16.54). If the interference cannot be avoided comfortably by mandibular displacement in chewing and swallowing by neuromuscular mechanisms (functional adaptation), if the tooth becomes mobile and is moved out of position (structural adaptation), and if the patient cannot ignore the discomfort or the presence of change for even a short period (behavioral adaptation), overt symptoms of dysfunction of the muscles, joints, periodontium, or teeth (pulp) may occur. However, such adaptive response and failure of adaptation are observed only rarely, and such observations do not qualify as

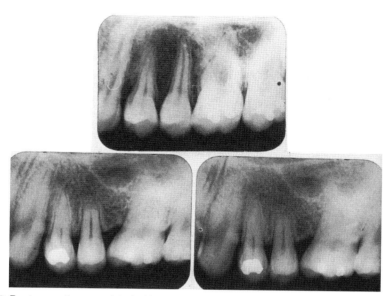

• **Fig. 16.52** Root resorption associated with high restoration and clenching habit. *Top,* Prior to placement of restoration. *Bottom left,* "Soreness" of the tooth began soon after the restoration and then rapidly some root resorption. High restoration was removed by selective grinding. *Bottom right,* Several months later, no evidence of soreness or additional root resorption.

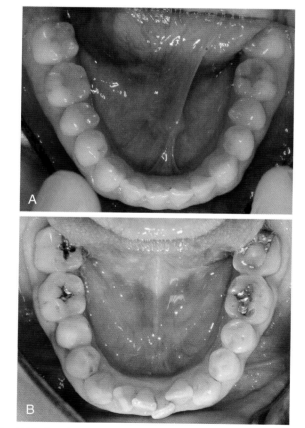

• **Fig. 16.53** Anterior crowding. (A) Absence of crowding. (B) Crowded mandibular incisors. Clinical findings of very tight proximal contacts and an occlusal interference in centric relation are only presumptive evidence of a cause-and-effect relationship between restorative treatment and anterior crowding.

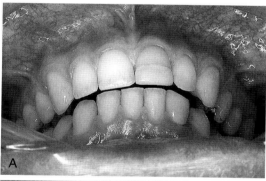

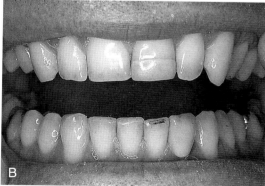

• **Fig. 16.54** Occlusal interference to closure in intercuspal position/centric occlusion due to restoration of the left maxillary central incisor. (A) Centric relation position. (B) Articulating paper mark on mandibular left lateral incisor. Temporomandibular disorder–like symptoms were relieved with adjustment of the centric occlusion interference.

scientific evidence. Models of research to test the validity of these clinical observations have serious flaws in design. Still, no clinician would knowingly put an occlusal interference in a restoration.

In addition to physical guidance from the teeth when the teeth are in contact during mastication or empty movements, mandibular guidance may occur before and during contact of the teeth from receptors in the periodontium and TMJs, and from other peripheral sensory receptors, as well as from higher centers in the central nervous system. It has been suggested that the anatomical relationships of the teeth and joints provide passive guidances and that active guidances involve reflexes originating in receptors in or around the teeth.[52] The question of feedback from various structures influencing mandibular movements and position is a complex one and cannot at this time be clearly answered.

The tendency to equate clinical responses with reflexes elicited under laboratory conditions rather than studying responses under natural conditions has led to what may be considered contradictory findings. It is also not unusual to find it assumed that failure to observe a response (i.e., a change in chewing patterns with anesthesia, occlusal interferences, and so on) is caused by the absence of a response rather than to a failure in the method of observation. Thus some responses may exist under natural conditions but have not been observed. Whether a changed anatomical feature of the occlusion causes an alteration of mandibular movement depends on a number of factors involving preprogramming, learning, adaptation or habituation, relationship to function and parafunction, and other central or peripheral influences.

Occlusal Interferences

In terms of clinical strategy, an occlusal contact relationship must interfere with something (e.g., function or parafunction) to be considered an occlusal interference (Fig. 16.55A and B). Thus a contact on the nonworking side is not an occlusal interference unless such a contact interferes with ongoing function and parafunction (i.e., prevents contact at some point on the working side).

In performing an indicated occlusal adjustment in centric relation, the clinician guides the jaw into a position of closure in a retruded contact position. In some individuals, premature occlusal contacts prevent a stable jaw relationship, and during guided rapid cyclical closure by the clinician, reflex jaw movements and muscle hyperactivity may occur to prevent such closure. Training of the patient and proper manipulation of the mandible in the absence of TMJ or muscle dysfunction may eliminate the muscle hyperactivity just long enough to guide the jaw into centric relation and to mark the occlusal interference with articulating paper (see Fig. 16.43). During the course of an occlusal adjustment to remove occlusal interferences to a stable occlusion in centric relation, a number of responses occur. For example, in some patients during the elimination of interferences, removal of a premature contact results in complete elimination of muscle resistance to guided jaw closure; that is, the clinician may close the jaw rapidly or slowly without any muscle response to prevent the closure. This may occur even with a slide in centric remaining, provided the contacts are bilateral and multiple, and freedom to move smoothly from centric relation to centric occlusion is possible.

Another clinical observation during the occlusal adjustment is that before eliminating a particular interference and before guiding the jaw into contact to determine whether that interference has been eliminated, all resistance and reflex muscle activity to prevent closure into the retruded contact position is gone. It should be kept in mind that during the course of an occlusal adjustment, a new but transient

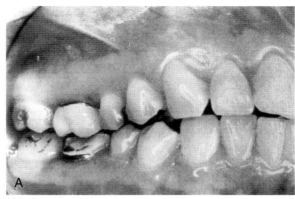

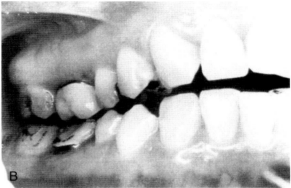

• **Fig. 16.55** Occlusal interference to function. (A) Intercuspal position. (B) Right working position of the mandible with interference by first molar restorations. Note absence of canine contact.

solitary occlusal interference may occur, or an interference may have greater significance for one tooth than another. These observations agree with the results of several studies showing that occlusal relations can lead to avoidance responses that probably serve to protect the teeth, muscles, joints, and periodontium from trauma because of occlusion. Training the patient to a hinge axis movement in the presence of occlusal interferences requires that no contact or anything even close to contact of the occlusion be made for several up-and-down movements and that the patient relax. Relaxation involves modulation of feedback from peripheral structures (joints, teeth, muscles, periodontium) and inhibitory effects from higher centers.

Vertical Dimension

Contact vertical dimension (occlusal vertical dimension) is the vertical component of the intercuspal position/centric occlusion. Although it would be helpful to be able to relate the contact relationship of the teeth to the rest position of the mandible (or the interocclusal space), optimal working length of the jaw elevator muscles, swallowing, speaking, or some other neurobehavioral parameter of function, vertical dimension is usually described in terms of the height of the lower third of the face, mandibular overclosure, or a need to "raise the bite" (increase the height of the teeth with restorations) because of worn-down or intruded posterior teeth (Fig. 16.56A) or impinging overbite (Fig. 16.56B). At present, no acceptable test of a presumed loss of vertical dimension appears available. The neurobehavioral aspects of the interocclusal space and occlusal vertical dimension are complex and require much further study.

It is not possible to determine with scientific assurance that aggressive bruxing and clenching in centric have caused intrusion

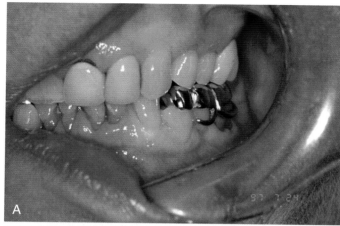

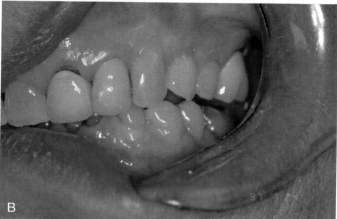

• **Fig. 16.56** Vertical dimension. (A) Use of a posterior bilateral onlay splint in an attempt to "raise the bite" and eliminate temporomandibular disorder symptoms. (B) An impinging overbite may require comprehensive orthodontics for correction, not an appliance as in (A).

or wear of the teeth or have been compensated for by eruption of the posterior teeth. Even short-term intrusion or loss of stops on posterior teeth may result in reflex-produced responses from anterior teeth because of premature contacts on anterior teeth. Again, no acceptable tests are available to determine with scientific assurance, even in the presence of dysfunction (e.g., temporomandibular disorder), that correction of a presumed loss of contact vertical dimension will correct the dysfunction.

Oral Motor Behavior

The term **oral motor behavior** is a convenience of speech that allows one to refer with a brief phrase to observable actions involving orofacial structures, including "simple" actions such as assumption of mandibular rest position and much more complex movements such as mastication. Human behavior reflects the translation of past, present, and ongoing ideas and learning (including sensations and emotions) into movements and actions. Although many of the responses or actions are common among all persons, the subjective response of a particular individual to a stimulus (including a change in the occlusion) may involve an inner experiential aspect of emotion in which the sensory experience may not fall into the usual acceptable range of pleasant or unpleasant. This aspect of sensation, referred to as **affect,** is the basis of much suffering and pleasure, including that related to the

occlusion and occlusal therapy. In mentalistic terms, feelings of pleasantness and unpleasantness are correlated with "motivation or intention to respond" and with emotion. Even a simple reflex may be considered as a unit of behavior. The advantage of viewing occlusion (in terms of function and parafunction) as human behavior is that the clinician has a better understanding of functional disturbances (e.g., TMJ, muscle disorders) and the recognition that how patients feel and respond to their occlusion is an important aspect of diagnosis and dental treatment.

Motivation

Emotion is a motivational phenomenon that plays a significant role in the determination of behavior. Motivation or drive and emotional states may be the basis for oral motor behavior, which is a fundamental component of ingestive responses, and for other behaviors essential for adaptation and survival. In effect, oral motor behavior can be initiated not only by situations involving cognitive processes but also by emotive processes, including homeostatic drives (e.g., hunger) concerned with the internal environment and nonhomeostatic drives (e.g., fear) related to adaptation to the external environment. The external environment may begin at the interface between oral sensory receptors and external stimuli involved in oral function and parafunction. However, ideas suggesting a "hard" interface between the internal and external environment are rapidly being reevaluated in terms of functional criteria. It is no longer possible to restrict thinking to a concept of the external environment as being "out there." From a psychophysiological standpoint, an interface between the external and internal worlds may not exist.

Homeostasis

As already indicated, oral motor behavior involves the translation of thought, sensation, and emotion into actions. Implied is the idea that actions or behavior may change because of learning and that some drive or motivation alters existing responses to environmental variables. Although the neural substrate for the translation of innate drives appears to exist, and regulatory behavior such as eating has clear value to the immediate survival of an individual, other oral motor behavior may not have clear antecedents in individual or group survival. However, during the development of the nervous system and motor functions, oral motor behavior may be highly dependent on homeostatic drives concerned with ingestive processes. Later oral motor behavior is an expression of the plasticity of the organism over a long period and consists of a whole complex of emotive and cognitive determinants that cannot be related easily to a hypothetical construct of homeostatic needs in the adult organism, even in a teleological sense.

Execution of Motor Behavior

Although oral motor behavior is judged on the basis of observable actions, the strategy and tactics of the occlusal aspects of human behavior are based on past dental experiences and the present state of the joints, muscles, periodontium, contact relation of the teeth, and central nervous system. The neural mechanisms that underlie the initiation, programming, and execution of motor behavior can be described only briefly here.

Complex behavior may involve neuronal circuits called **pattern generators,** which, when activated, elicit stereotyped, rhythmic, and/or coordinated movements. The pattern generators for locomotion appear to be in the spinal cord and to be activated by discrete nuclei or regions in the brainstem, and they can be accessed by higher-level structures in the central nervous system. The pattern generators for chewing and swallowing are located in the brainstem medullary-pontine reticular formation. As already mentioned, limbic structures appear to have access to pattern generators.

Chewing is a type of oral motor behavior that demonstrates centrally programmed movement and in part peripherally driven movement. Controlled interaction is more often the case than either purely centrally programmed movement or purely peripherally controlled movement. Pattern generators may be part of the particular programs accessed by higher brain centers to generate complex behavior.

Swallowing

Swallowing involves the coordination of almost 20 different muscles with motor neurons distributed from mesencephalic to posterior medullary levels. The patterning of muscular contractions is independent of the stimulus necessary to evoke swallowing. The neurons responsible for coordination include a **swallowing center,** in which neuronal groups fire automatically in a particular sequence when stimulated to achieve the necessary pattern of muscle activity to produce swallowing. "Triggering," or initiation of a central program, involves neurons in the motor cortex that act as command elements and control patterns of neuronal activity as well as receive feedback from the systems controlled. Thus movement may be centrally programmed (drive) and at the same time modulated by peripheral influences.

The cyclical movements of the jaw in mastication reflect past experiences, adaptive behavior, neuronal activity of the mesencephalic rhythm generator and the trigeminal motor nucleus, and the influence of oral reflexes, either conditioned or unconditioned. The pattern generator may be influenced by sensory input from the orofacial area and influences from higher centers in the central nervous system.

Summary

To understand occlusion in its broadest sense, it is necessary to consider, in addition to TMJ articulation, muscles, and teeth, some of the neurobehavioral mechanisms that give meaning to the presence and function of the masticatory system. Although many of the neural mechanisms mediating interaction between occlusion and thoughts, sensations, and emotions are complex and often indeterminate, it is possible to suggest strategies that could account for the variety of responses (physiological and psychological) that occur in function and parafunction.

The "obvious" strategy to compensate for wear of proximal contact areas is mesial migration of the teeth, and the strategy to compensate for wear of the occlusal surfaces is eruption of the teeth. The strategy for regulating the contraction of the jaw elevators to achieve a normal resting position of the mandible with a small interocclusal space is a postural reflex (stretch reflex). The overall strategy for motivation to have access to the muscles of mastication might be to provide a drive for ingestive processes, especially during the early stages of development of the masticatory system and maturation of the nervous system—swallowing in fetal life, suckling in the newborn, and chewing in the young infant.

It appears plausible, at least, that emotion may be important not only as a motivational phenomenon but also as a reflection of what is agreeable or disagreeable about something that is placed in the mouth, including items not considered to be food and perhaps even restorations that interfere with function or parafunction. Demonstration of evidence for and against strategies to explain completely neurobehavioral mechanisms of "occlusion" requires much more space than provided here.

The extensive "education" of persons through the television media, newspapers, magazines, and the internet and through professional dental care and instructions to patients not only has produced an awareness of the teeth and mouth but also has coupled these structures to a sense of health and comfort. The affect involved in such a sense of well-being about oral health involves part of the same neurobehavioral substrate underlying innate drives, motivation, and emotional states necessary for biological adaptation and survival of the species. Ingestive processes, which include oral motor responses involved in mastication, are essential for survival. Functional disturbances of the masticatory system may involve psychophysiological mechanisms that are related to the teeth and their functions. Therefore occlusal interferences to function or parafunction may then involve more than simply contact relations of the teeth; they may involve psychophysiological mechanisms of human behavior as well.

No scientific evidence is available for making a specific structure or psychophysiological mechanism the sole cause of TMJ/muscle dysfunction. However, any attempt to negate the role of the teeth in human behavior, including dysfunction, perhaps is made by those who have not had the opportunity to observe the effect on affect, favorable neuromuscular response, and elimination of discomfort when appropriate occlusal therapy is rendered.

Unfortunately, neuroscientific evidence to separate the subjective from objective clinical observations has not lived up to its full potential. Scientific clinical studies in which true cause-and-effect relationships can be determined are difficult to design, especially when such relationships may be indirect, "on-again, off-again," and significantly influenced by the observer and other factors under natural conditions.[52] Considerably more appropriate research is needed to establish the role of occlusion and related factors in TMJ/muscle dysfunction.

Pretest Answers

1. C
2. A
3. A
4. C
5. B

References

1. Zwemer TJ: *Mosby's dental dictionary*, St Louis, 1998, Mosby.
2. Ash MM, Ramfjord SP: *Occlusion*, ed 4, Philadelphia, 1995, Saunders.
3. Angle EH: In *The angle system of regulation and retention of the teeth*, Philadelphia, 1887, S.S. White Dental Manufacturing.
4. Schuyler CH: Principles employed in full denture prostheses which may be applied to other fields of dentistry, *J Am Dent Assoc* 16:2045, 1929.
5. Beyron HL: Characteristics of functionally optimal occlusion and principles of occlusal rehabilitation, *J Am Dent Assoc* 48:648, 1954.
6. D'Amico A: The canine teeth—normal functional relation of the natural teeth in man, *J South Calif Dent Assoc* 1:6–23, 1958. 2:49–60; 4:127–142; 5:175–182; 6:194–208; 7:239–241.
7. Friel S: The development of ideal occlusion of the gum pads and teeth, *Am J Orthod* 40:1963, 1954.

5. Misch CE: *Contemporary implant dentistry*, ed 3, St Louis, 2008, Mosby.
6. Gladwin MA, Bagby M: *Clinical aspects of dental materials*, ed 3, Baltimore, 2009, Lippincott Williams & Wilkins.
7. Rosenstiel SF, Land MF, Fujimoto J: *Contemporary fixed prosthodontics*, ed 4, St Louis, 2006, Mosby.
8. Zarb GA, Bolender CL: *Prosthodontic treatment for edentulous patients*, ed 12, St Louis, 2004, Mosby.
9. Page D: Digital radiography in forensic odontology, *Forensic Magazine,* 2005. http://www.forensicmag.com/articles/2005/04/digital-radiography-forensic-odontology#.Upex1Cfzi1A.
10. Stephan CN, Simpson EK: Facial soft tissue depths in craniofacial identification part I: an analytical review of the published adult data, *J Forensic Sci* 53(6):1257, 2008.
11. Wang Y, et al.: Non-negative matrix factorization framework for face recognition, *Int J Pattern Recogn Artif Intell* 194:495, 2005.
12. Bitemarks. www.forensicmed.co.uk/wounds/bitemarks/?utm_source=paste&utm_campaign=copypaste&utm_cor.
13. Hupp JR, Ellis E, Tucker R: *Contemporary oral and maxillofacial surgery*, ed 5, St Louis, 2008, Mosby.
14. Pappalardo S, Guarnieri R: Randomized clinical study comparing piezosurgery and conventional surgery in mandibular cyst enucleation, *J Craniomaxillofac Surg* 6:186, 2013.
15. Chrcanovic BR, Freire-Maia B: Considerations of maxillary tuberosity fractures during extraction of upper molars: a literature review, *Dental Traumatology* 5:393, 2011.
16. Nield-Gehrig JS: *Fundamentals of periodontal instrumentation & advanced root instrumentation*, ed 6, Baltimore, 2008, Lippincott Williams & Wilkins.
17. Versianiet MA, et al.: Enamel pearls in permanent dentition: case report and micro-CT evaluation, *Dentomaxillofacial Radiology* 426:20120332, 2013.
18. Newman MG, et al.: *Carranza's clinical periodontology*, ed 11, St Louis, 2012, Saunders.
19. Rose LF, et al.: *Periodontics medicine, surgery, and implants*, St Louis, 2004, Mosby.
20. Stock CJ, Walker RT, Gulabivala K: *Endodontics*, ed 3, Edinburgh, 2004, Mosby.
21. Torabinejad M, Walton RE: *Endodontics principles and practice*, ed 4, St Louis, 2009, Saunders.
22. Krishnan IS, Sreedharan SA: Comparative evaluation of electronic and radiographic determination of root canal length in primary teeth: an in vitro study, *Contemp Clin Dent* 34:416, 2012.
23. Gordon MP, Chandler NP: Electronic apex locators, *Int Endod J* 386:417, 2005.
24. Connert T, et al.: Accuracy of endodontic working length determination using cone beam computed tomography, *Int Endod J* 18, 2013.
25. Niazi SA, et al.: The effectiveness of enzymic irrigation in removing a nutrient-stressed endodontic multi-species biofilm, *Int Endod J* 18, 2013.
26. Kalwar A, et al.: The efficiency of root canal disinfection using a diode laser: in vitro study, *Indian J Dent Res* 241:14, 2013.
27. Friedlander LT, Cullinan MP, Love RM: Dental stem cells and their potential role in apexogensis and apexification, *Int Endod J* 4211:955, 2009.
28. Bansal R, Bansal R: Regenerative endodontics: a state of the art, *Indian J Dent Res* 221:122, 2011.
29. Honda MJ, et al.: Mesenchymal dental stem cells for tissue regeneration, *Int J Oral Maxillofac Implants* 286:e451, 2013.
30. Roberson T, Heymann HO, Swift EJ: *Sturdevant's art and science of operative dentistry*, ed 5, St Louis, 2006, Mosby.
31. Summitt JB, et al.: *Fundamentals of operative dentistry*, ed 3, Chicago, 2006, Quintessence Publishing Co.
32. Pinkham J, et al.: *Pediatric dentistry: infancy through adolescence*, ed 4, St Louis, 2005, Saunders.
33. Shillingburg HT, et al.: *Fundamentals of fixed prosthodontics*, ed 3, Carol Stream, 1997, Quintessence Publishing Co.
34. Chiche G, Pinault A: *Esthetics of anterior fixed prosthodontics*, Chicago, 1994, Quintessence Publishing Co.
35. Frese C, Staehle HJ, Wolff D: The assessment of dentofacial esthetics in restorative dentistry: a review of the literature, *J Am Dent Assoc* 1435:461, 2012.
36. Witt M, Flores-Mir C: Laypeople's preference regarding frontal dentofacial esthetics: periodontal factors, *J Am Dent Assoc* 1428:925, 2011.
37. Raj V: Esthetic paradigms in the interdisciplinary management of maxillary anterior dentition—a review, *J Esthet Restor Dent* 255:295, 2013.
38. Dorfman W, Dossetter DS: *The smile guide*, Los Angeles, 2004, Discus Dental, Inc.
39. Golub-Evans J: Unity and variety: essential ingredients of a smile design, *Current Opinion in Cosmetic Dentistry*, 1, 1994.
40. Okeson JP: *Management of temporomandibular disorders and occlusion*, ed 6, St Louis, 2008, Mosby.
41. Bhusari P, et al.: Prevalence of enamel projections and its co-relation with furcation involvement in maxillary and mandibular molars: a study on dry skull, *J Indian Soc Periodontol* 175:601, 2013.
42. Kulkarni VK, et al.: Endodontic treatment and esthetic management of a primary double tooth with direct composite using silicone buildup guide, *Contemp Clin Dent* 3(Suppl 1):S92, 2012.
43. Spencer J, et al.: Special consideration regarding the assessment and management of patients being treated with mandibular advancement oral appliance therapy for snoring and obstructive sleep apnea, *Cranio* 311:10, 2013.
44. Ash M, Ramfjord SP: *Occlusion*, ed 4, St Louis, 1995, Saunders.
45. Nelson SJ: Principles of stabilization bite splint therapy, *Dent Clin North Am* 39:403, 1995.
46. Okeson JP: *Management of temporomandibular disorders and occlusion*, ed 7, St Louis, 2013, Mosby.

Appendix A

Review of Tooth Morphology

Appendix A includes color renditions of Figures 2.3 and 2.4 considered in Chapter 2 on the eruption and development of the teeth. They can be used to demonstrate to patients the development of the dentitions from 5 months in utero to adolescence and adulthood.

Also included are representative views of the facial/labial/buccal and occlusal/incisal aspects of all of the teeth considered in Chapters 6 through 12. Because of the proximity of these illustrations to the traits and characteristics of the teeth provided in Appendix B, page turns to earlier chapters can be minimized. It is also possible to view these same illustrations on the Evolve site while examining the traits and characteristics in Appendix B.

DECIDUOUS DENTITION

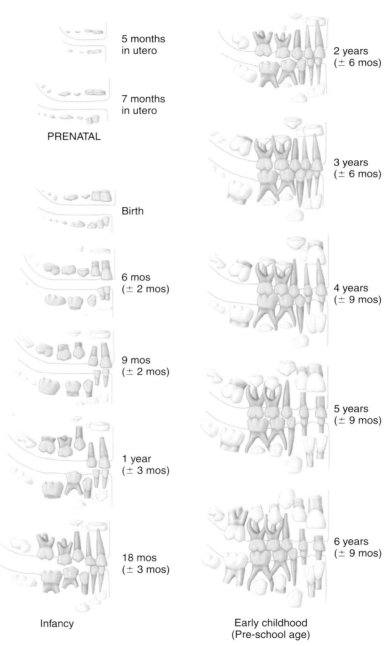

5 months
in utero

7 months
in utero

PRENATAL

Birth

6 mos
(± 2 mos)

9 mos
(± 2 mos)

1 year
(± 3 mos)

18 mos
(± 3 mos)

Infancy

2 years
(± 6 mos)

3 years
(± 6 mos)

4 years
(± 9 mos)

5 years
(± 9 mos)

6 years
(± 9 mos)

Early childhood
(Pre-school age)

• **Appendix A.1** Development of the human dentition to the sixth year. The primary teeth are the blue ones in the illustration. (Modified from Schour, L. & Massler, M. [1941]. The development of the human dentition, *J Am Dent Assoc, 28,* 1153.)

MIXED DENTITION   PERMANENT DENTITION

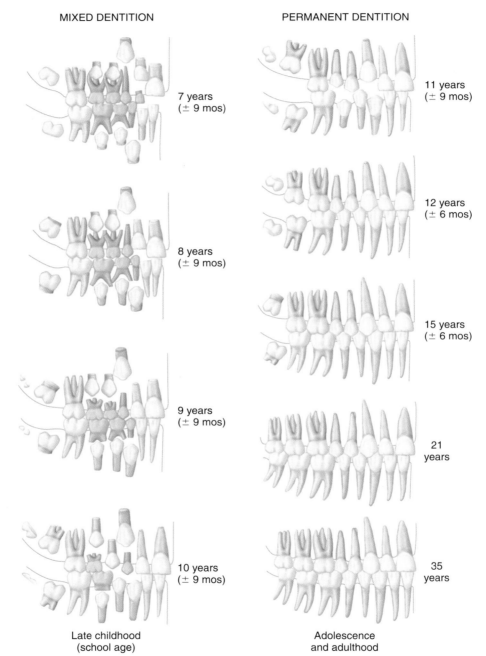

7 years
(± 9 mos)

11 years
(± 9 mos)

8 years
(± 9 mos)

12 years
(± 6 mos)

9 years
(± 9 mos)

15 years
(± 6 mos)

10 years
(± 9 mos)

21
years

35
years

Late childhood
(school age)

Adolescence
and adulthood

• **Appendix A.2** Development of the human dentition from the seventh year to maturity. Note the displacement of the primary teeth. (Modified from Schour, L. & Massler, M. [1941]. The development of the human dentition, *J Am Dent Assoc, 28,* 1153.)

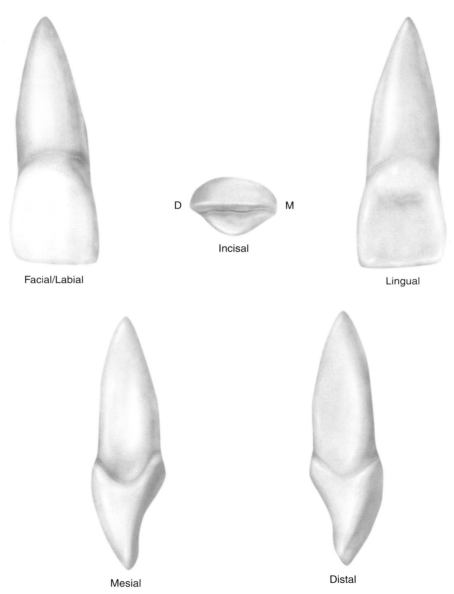

Facial/Labial

D M

Incisal

Lingual

Mesial

Distal

• **Appendix A.3** Maxillary central incisor (right).

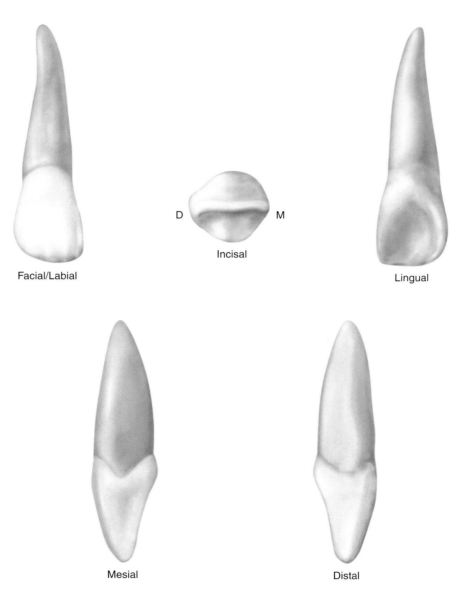

Facial/Labial

Incisal

D   M

Lingual

Mesial

Distal

• **Appendix A.4** Maxillary lateral incisor (right).

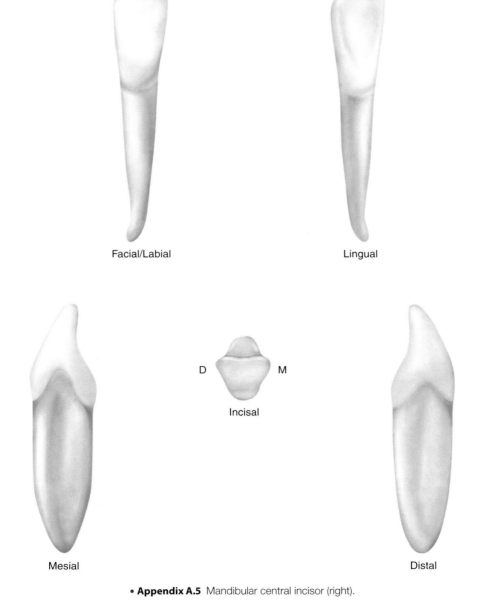

Facial/Labial

Lingual

D   M

Incisal

Mesial

Distal

• **Appendix A.5** Mandibular central incisor (right).

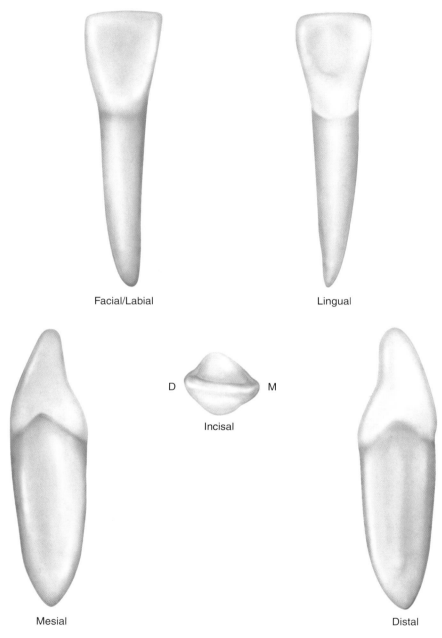

Facial/Labial

Lingual

D ⌢ M

Incisal

Mesial

Distal

• **Appendix A.6** Mandibular lateral incisor (right).

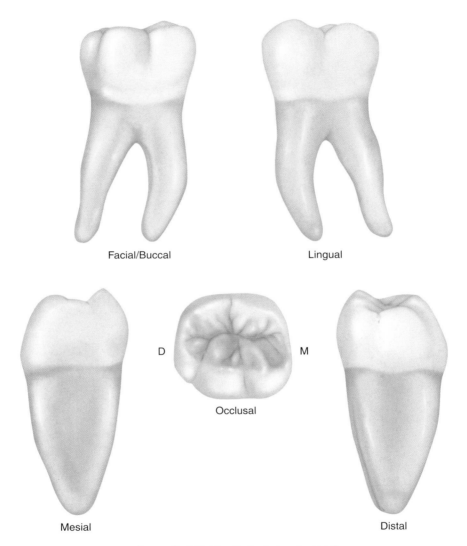

Facial/Buccal

Lingual

D

M

Occlusal

Mesial

Distal

• **Appendix A.15** Mandibular first molar (right).

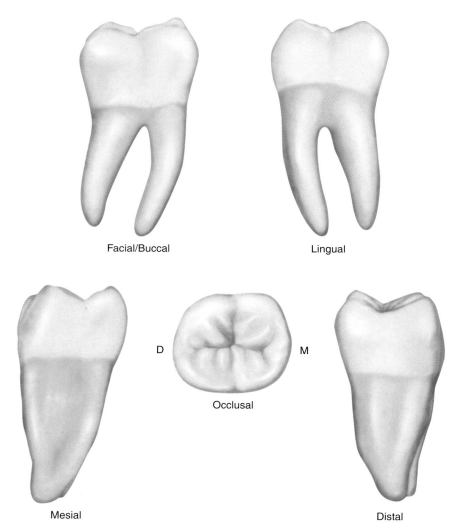

Facial/Buccal

Lingual

D

M

Occlusal

Mesial

Distal

• **Appendix A.16** Mandibular second molar (right).

Appendix B

Tooth Traits of the Permanent Dentition

Appendix B includes tables listing important traits and characteristics of the teeth in the permanent dentition. The tables can be used in conjunction with the illustrations in Appendix A to note differences and similarities in tooth morphology. Tooth notation systems, dimensions, position of proximal contacts, heights of contour, curvature of the cementoenamel junction, and features of various profile, incisal, and occlusal views are summarized to facilitate the study of dental anatomy.

TABLE 1   Maxillary Incisors: Type Traits and Other Characteristics

	Central Incisor	Lateral Incisor
Facial/Labial Aspect	Fig. 6.9	Fig. 6.19
Proximal contacts	Cervico-incisal location	—
Mesial	Incisal third	Junction incisal/middle thirds
Distal	Junction incisal/middle thirds	Middle third
Mesioincisal angle	Sharp right angle	Slightly rounded
Distoincisal angle	Slightly rounded	Distinctly rounded
Mesial profile	Straight	Slightly rounded
Distal profile	Nearly round	Distinctly rounded
Mesiodistal width	Comparatively wide	Comparatively narrow
Pulp horn(s)	3 (facial view)	Usually 2 (facial view)
Lobes	4 (Fig. 4.12, *A*)	4
Lingual Aspect	Fig. 6.3	Fig. 6.14
Marginal ridges	Moderate	More prominent
Cingulum	Moderately pronounced	More prominent
Fossa	Moderately deep	Deep
Incisal Aspect	Fig. 6.11	Fig. 6.18
Outline	Triangular	Ovoid
Labial	Slightly convex	More convex
Dimensions	Table 6.1	Table 6.2
Crown length (cervico-incisal)	10.5 mm	9 mm
Crown diameter		
Mesiodistal	8.5 mm	6.5 mm
Cervical	7.0 mm	5.0 mm
Labiolingual	7.0 mm	6.0 mm
Contour height	0.5 mm; Figs. 6.4, 6.5	0.5 mm; Fig. 6.13
Facial/lingual	Both cervical third	Both cervical third
Curvature at CEJ	Table 6.1	Table 6.2
Mesial	3.5 mm	3.0 mm
Distal	2.5 mm	2.0 mm
Root	Figs. 6.3, 6.5, 6.9, 6.10	Figs. 6.13, 6.19, 6.20
Length	13.0 mm	13.0 mm
Pulp canal(s)	1	Less frequent apical accessory canals
Chronology	Tables 2.3, 6.1	Tables 2.3, 6.2
Eruption	7–8 yr	8–9 yr
Root completed	10 yr	11 yr
Tooth Notations	Chapter 1	Chapter 1
Universal	Right: 8; left: 9	Right: 7; left: 10
International (FDI)	Right: 11; left: 21	Right: 12; left: 22
Palmer	Right/left: 1⌋ ⌊1	Right/left: 2⌋ ⌊2

TABLE 2   **Mandibular Incisors: Type Traits and Other Characteristics**

	Central Incisor	Lateral Incisor
Facial/Labial Aspect	Figs. 7.2, 7.9	Figs. 7.13, 7.19
Symmetry	Symmetrical bilaterally	Asymmetrical
Proximal contacts	Fig. 5.8, *A*	Fig. 5.8, *B*
Mesial	Incisal third	Incisal third
Distal	Incisal third	Incisal third
Mesioincisal angles	Sharp right angles	Some rounding
Distoincisal angles	Sharp right angles	More rounded than mesioincisal angle
Curvature at CEJ	Fig. 5.27, Table 7.1	Table 7.2
Mesial	3.0 mm	3.0 mm
Distal	2.0 mm	2.0 mm
Incisal Aspect	Fig. 7.11	Fig. 7.18
Incisal edge (ridge)	Right angle to line bisecting cingulum	Distolingual twist to line bisecting cingulum
Pulp horn(s)	1 or 0	Variable; more prominent
Lobes	4	4
Dimensions	Table 7.1	Table 7.2
Crown length (cervico-incisal)	9.5 mm	9.5 mm
Crown diameter		
Mesiodistal	5 mm	5.5 mm
Cervical	3.5 mm	4.0 mm
Labiolingual	6.0 mm	6.5 mm
Contour height	Less than 0.5 mm; Fig. 7.7	Less than 0.5 mm
Facial/lingual	Both cervical third	Both cervical third
Root		
Dimensions	Table 7.1	Table 7.2
Length	12.5 mm	14.0 mm
Pulp (root) canal(s)	Usually 1; 2 possible	1
Chronology	Table 7.1	Table 7.2
Eruption	6–7 yr	7–8 yr
Root completed	9 yr	10 yr
Tooth Notations	Chapter 1	Chapter 1
Universal	Right: 25; left: 24	Right: 26; left: 23
International (FDI)	Right: 41; left: 31	Right: 42; left: 32
Palmer	Right/left: 1̅ ⌐1	Right/left: 2̅ ⌐2

TABLE 3 Maxillary and Mandibular Incisors: Arch Traits and Other Characteristics

Maxillary Incisors	Mandibular Incisors
Central incisor wider than lateral incisor	Lateral incisor wider than central incisor
Wider than mandibular central incisor	Narrowest of incisor class
Marginal ridges and cingulum more prominent	Marginal ridges and cingulum not prominent
Lingual fossa pronounced, often with a lingual pit	Lingual fossa shallow without grooves or pits
Crown width greater mesiodistally than labiolingually	Crown width greater labiolingually than mesiodistally
Roots rounded in cross section	Roots thin mesiodistally
Incisal edge labial to root axis	Incisal edge lingual to root axis

TABLE 4 Canines: Type and Arch Traits and Other Characteristics

	Maxillary Canine	Mandibular Canine
Facial/Labial Aspect		
Proximal contacts	Fig. 5.8, *C*	Fig. 5.7, *C*
Mesial	Junction incisal/middle thirds	Incisal third
Distal	Middle third	Middle third
Mesial Aspect	Wider faciolingually	Narrower, longer
Lingual Aspect	Deeper lingual fossae	Flat lingual surface
Marginal ridges	Pronounced; 2 fossae	Parallel or slightly converging
Cingulum	Large, centered mesiodistally	Smaller, may be off center distally
Lingual pits, grooves	Common	None
Incisal Aspect	Marked asymmetry of mesial/distal halves	Less symmetry; distal cusp ridge rotated
Incisal/Proximal Aspects	Cusp tip may be at or labial to root axis line	Cusp tip lingual to root axis line
Dimensions		
Mesiodistal	7.5 mm	7.0 mm
Labiolingual	8.0 mm	7.5 mm
Curvature at CEJ	2.5 mm (mesial)	1.0 mm (distal)
Incisal-cervical	10.0 mm	11.0 mm
Contour height	0.5 mm	Less than 0.5 mm
Facial/lingual	Both cervical third	Both cervical third
Pulp horn(s)	1	1
Lobes	4	4
Root		
Terminal (number)	1	Maybe 2 (Fig. 8.24)
Length	17 mm	16 mm
Chronology	Table 8.1	Table 8.2
Eruption	11–12 yr	9–10 yr
Root completed	13–15 yr	12–14 yr
Tooth Notations	Chapter 1	Chapter 1
Universal	Right: 6; left: 11	Right: 27; left: 22
International (FDI)	Right: 13; left: 23	Right: 43; left: 33
Palmer	Right/left: 3⌋ ⌊3	Right/left: 3⌋ ⌊3

TABLE 5   Maxillary Premolars: Type Traits and Other Characteristics

	First Premolar	Second Premolar
Facial/Buccal Aspect		
Proximal contacts	Mesial/distal: middle third	Mesial/distal: middle third
Shoulders	Prominent	Narrow
Buccal cusp	Tipped more to distal	Not tipped
Cusp ridges	Longer mesial ridge	Similar
Cusp size, height	Slightly wider, longer	Shorter
Lingual Aspect	Buccal profile visible	Profile not visible
Mesial Aspect		
Mesiomarginal groove	Crosses marginal ridge	Does not cross ridge
Mesial concavity	Present	Not present
Mesial root depression	Present	Present
Occlusal Aspect	Fig. 9.6	Fig. 9.21
Profile	Hexagonal	Ovoid
Central groove	Long	Short
Supplemental groves	Usually not present	Many; often present
Lobes	4	4
Pulp horn(s)	2	2
Dimensions	Table 9.1	Table 9.2
Cervico-occlusal	8.5 mm	8.5 mm
Crown diameter		
Mesiodistal	7.0 mm	7.0 mm
Cervical	5.0 mm	5.0 mm
Buccolingual	9.0 mm	9.0 mm
Contour height	Fig. 9.5	Fig. 9.19
Facial/buccal crest	Cervical third	Cervical third
Lingual	Middle third	Middle third
Curvature at CEJ	Figs. 9.4, 9.5	
Mesial	1.0 mm	1.0 mm
Distal	0.0 mm	0.0 mm
Root		
Length of root	14.0 mm	14.0 mm
Grooves	Distinct, longitudinal	No distinct grooves
Number of roots	Usually 2	1 root
Pulp canal(s)	Often 2	Usually 1
Chronology	Table 9.1	Table 9.2
Eruption	10–11 yr	10–12 yr
Root completed	12–13 yr	12–14 yr
Tooth Notations	Chapter 1	Chapter 1
Universal	Right, 5; left, 12	Right, 4; left, 13
International (FDI)	Right, 14; left, 24	Right, 15; left, 25
Palmer	Right/left: 4⌋ ⌊4	Right/left: 5⌋ ⌊5

TABLE 6   Mandibular Premolars: Type Traits and Other Characteristics

	First Premolar	Second Premolar
Facial/Buccal Aspect	Figs. 10.2, 10.9	Figs. 10.13, 10.18
Proximal contacts	Fig. 5.7	Fig. 5.7
Cervico-occlusal	Mesial/distal: middle third	Mesial/distal: middle third
Form	Asymmetrical	Bilaterally symmetrical
Lingual Aspect	Fig. 10.3	Fig. 10.14
Buccal profile	All buccal profile seen	None seen
Cusp height	Lingual less than buccal	Buccal/lingual cusps nearly equal
Mesial Aspect	Fig. 10.1	Fig. 10.15
Occlusal plane	Tilted lingually	Essentially horizontal
Transverse ridge or buccal triangular ridge	Transverse ridge present (Fig. 10.1)	No transverse ridge present (Fig. 10.17)
Occlusal Aspect	Figs. 10.6, 10.11	Fig. 10.17
Outline form	Diamond-shaped	Square
Cusps	2 (Fig. 10.1)	2 or 3 (Fig. 10.20)
Lobes	4	4 or 5
Dimensions	Table 10.1	Table 10.2
Crown length (cervico-occlusal)	8.5 mm	8.0 mm
Crown diameter		
Mesiodistal	7.0 mm	7.0 mm
Cervical	5.0 mm	5.0 mm
Buccolingual	7.5 mm	8.0 mm
Contour height	Figs. 5.27, 10.4	Fig. 10.16
Facial	Cervical third	Middle third
Lingual	Middle third	Middle third
Curvature at CEJ	Table 10.1 (cervical line)	Table 10.2
Mesial	1.0 mm	1.0 mm
Distal	0.0 mm	0.0 mm
Root	Table 10.1	Table 10.2
Length	14.0 mm	14.5 mm
Pulp canal(s)	1	1
Pulp horn(s)	1	2
Chronology	Table 2.3; Table 10.1	Table 2.3; Table 10.2
Eruption	10–12 yr	11–12 yr
Root completed	12–13 yr	13–14 yr
Tooth Notations	Chapter 1	Chapter 1
Universal	Right: 28; left: 21	Right: 29; left: 20
International (FDI)	Right: 44; left: 34	Right: 45; left: 35
Palmer	Right/left: 4⌐ ⌐4	Right/left: 5⌐ ⌐5

TABLE 7   Premolars: Arch Traits and Other Characteristics

Maxillary Premolars	Mandibular Premolars
Facial/Buccal Aspect: Fig. 4.16	
Crowns are trapezoidal*	Crowns are trapezoidal
Mesial Aspect: Fig. 4.16	
Crowns are trapezoidal	Crowns are rhomboidal†
Buccal and lingual cusps are almost equal in height	Lingual cusps comparatively much shorter than maxillary lingual cusps Lingual cusp tips may be lingual to the root
Two major cusps of almost equal size and prominence	Buccal and lingual cusps of uneven height and prominence

*A trapezoid is a four-sided plane figure having two sides parallel.
†A rhomboid is an oblique-angled parallelogram with only the opposite sides equal.